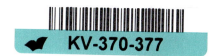

GOOD HOUSEKEEPING
GUIDE TO
MEDICINES

GOOD HOUSEKEEPING
GUIDE TO
MEDICINES

Dr. Eric Trimmer

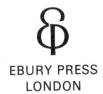

EBURY PRESS
LONDON

Published by Ebury Press
National Magazine House
72 Broadwick Street
London W1V 2BP

First impression 1983

ISBN 0 85223 269 1 (hardback)
ISBN 0 85223 211 X (paperback)

Designed by Harry Green
Typeset by Advanced Filmsetters (Glasgow) Ltd
Printed and Bound in Italy by New Interlitho SPA, Milan

TABLE OF
CONTENTS

Introduction: Why this book?   9

1 Treatment for problems involving the mouth, stomach and bowels   14
The mouth and gums · The gullet (oesophagus) and the problems of hiatus
hernia · The treatment of dyspepsia, peptic ulcers and gastrointestinal spasm
The kinds of diarrhoeas · Remedies for constipation

2 Treatments used for problems involving the chest and breathing   37
Remedies that help wheezing · The prevention of asthma · Cough mixtures

3 Remedies that suppress the appetite   53
Compound slimming remedies · Slimming 'specialities'

4 Remedies for control of infection   58
The penicillins · The cephalosporins · The tetracyclines · Other antibiotics
The sulphonamides and co-trimoxazole · Treating tuberculosis · Fungal
infection treatment · The development of drugs active against viruses

5 Treating diseases of the thyroid function   72
Thyroid deficiency disease · Overaction of the thyroid gland

6 Remedies used for the skin   76
Skin cleaning, shampoos and antiseptics · Skin infections and their treatment
Skin protection and camouflage · Anti-itch (antipruritic) preparations
Acne medications · Warts, corns and calluses · Eczema and psoriasis
treatments

7 Treating disorders of sexual function   98
Remedies for infertility: the male · Remedies for infertility: the female
Management of the menopause · Treatment of sexual problems · Remedies
used to treat hypersexuality

8 Remedies used to overcome worm infestations   105
Threadworm remedies · Roundworm remedies · Hookworm remedies
Tapeworm remedies · Multiple worm infestation remedies

9 Contraception 109
Contraception for the male—the condom · Contraception for the female

10 Managing anaemia 117
The rationale of iron replacement therapy · Treatment for anaemia caused by iron and folic acid deficiency in pregnancy · Compound iron preparations

11 Remedies for rheumatism 123
Managing 'rheumatic' arthritis · Treatment for gout · Other treatment of rheumatism

12 Remedies for nausea and giddiness 132
Motion sickness and its treatment · Pregnancy sickness and its treatment Vomiting secondary to illness · Dizziness (giddiness, vertigo)

13 Remedies that act on the eye 136
Remedies used to combat infection · Steroid preparations · Other eye-drops for inflammation and allergy · The management of glaucoma · Other eye problems

14 The problems of the ear, nose, mouth and throat and their treatment 144
The ear · The nose (obstructed and streaming) · General flu remedies General mouth and throat problems

15 Treating problems of the nerves 153
Drugs that sedate, control anxiety and promote sleep · Treating psychosis and related illnesses (including depression, mania, schizophrenia) · The control of epilepsy · Treating Parkinson's disease · Drugs used for choreas, tics and related disorders

16 Remedies that control pain 177
General pain control—mild to moderate, and severe pain control · Migraine remedies · Remedies used for trigeminal neuralgia · Remedies for pain arising in the urinary tract · Compound analgesics

Appendix—Drug interaction 193

General Index—Diseases and conditions 196

Drug index and list 198

TO EVERYONE
USING THIS BOOK

The precautions, dosages and side effects quoted in this book are based on current medical knowledge, together with my own experience as a doctor and as a medical journalist. However, anyone who finds that the information given here differs materially from that contained on a prescription, or who experiences unusual or extreme side effects, should consult his GP and/or local pharmacist immediately.

ACKNOWLEDGEMENTS

The production of this book has only been possible by frequent reference to standard works and text books. *The Pharmacological Basis of Therapeutics* by Louis S. Goodman and Alfred Gilman has been constantly at my side. *The British National Formulary*, the *Monthly Index of Medical Specialities* (MIMS) and the *ABPI Data Sheet Compendium* have both been invaluable. In the very difficult area of drugs available over-the-counter at the chemist's ▲ (OTC), I have received invaluable advice from Stan Gottlieb, B.Pharm MPS, who has prevented many a potential gaffe and who, together with my secretary, Jane Foley, has battled worthily with difficult subject matter and helped enormously in many ways.

ERIC TRIMMER *London 1983*

WHY THIS BOOK?

The first reason

Statistics tell us that the chances are you will be taking something in the way of a medicine within a very little while of reading this. Exactly what you are taking will, of course, vary. It may be something you've bought over the counter at the chemist's for a headache or indigestion. The use of these OTC remedies, as they are now called, is much more prevalent these days than earlier. This does not mean that we are becoming a race of hypochondriacs, but merely that most OTC remedies are very good and efficient. The majority are produced by large pharmaceutical manufacturers that, anyway, make the medicines that doctors prescribe. Their quality control is excellent and, properly used, they are extremely safe. Because they *are* so efficient more folk would rather swallow a few pills to chase away a headache than put up with the pain and discomfort. Or take a dose of this or that to stop the worst symptoms of a streaming cold or, for that matter, a painful menstrual period.

Of course the chemist; or even his assistant, will often be helpful in suggesting a medicine for your symptoms—and let's be realistic, getting rid of symptoms is really what you are after. In the past doctors have shaken their heads about this 'symptomatic' treatment, as they call it. They point out that symptoms are there for a reason, as a warning, and to help with diagnosis of a disease. Today, I think, the medical profession has moved from this somewhat arbitrary and restrictive attitude. Doctors themselves now rely heavily on 'symptomatic' treatment when they prescribe, and the reason for this is not hard to fathom. In many cases it is the only treatment they have—say for colds, flu and many other ills that plague us.

What we are really saying is this. A great many episodes of illness are 'self-limiting'. They will get better by themselves. Unless this was so the whole human race would have died out years ago instead of multiplying to fill the earth. But many of these 'self-limiting' diseases are extremely unpleasant while you are actually suffering them. A boil on the back of someone's neck can be an object of fun—except when that neck is yours. A short sharp attack of fibrositis or lumbago may raise a smile when you see your neighbour hobbling around like an old man—but when you get an attack of the 'screws' or whatever they call it down your way, the chances are you won't want to soldier on until Nature in her quiet, but often long-winded way, produces the cure. So you decide to take something—and fast.

This is a very sensible attitude and, as we've said, the expert advice you can get at a chemist is invaluable. But very often you don't get your OTC medication at the chemist. Perhaps there is already something in your medicine chest at home that looks as though it would do the trick. Maybe your husband's back ache would respond to the tablets you found so helpful with your painful periods. You could be right in such a case—but you might also be terribly wrong. This is one of the things this book will tell you—how not to make matters worse by taking the *wrong* medicine. By guiding you along the right road in selecting an effective remedy for your everyday illnesses, it will help you and yours to get better quickly and safely.

For years now there has been a sort of 'dark ages' conspiracy about the sensible self-selection of helpful treatments by the public—and I suspect it has been carefully fostered by elements within the medical profession who fear that their 'secrets' are too powerful to be shared or trusted to others. The mystery must be protected they feel, or the 'magic' will slowly disappear. Strangely perhaps, one branch of medicine—homoeopathy—has always been very open in this way. It has encouraged its clientele to become familiar with a few suitable remedies to help with the problems of living. In orthodox medicine too, there are signs of change on this score, and more and more doctors are encouraging people to use the chemist more often and more intelligently.

There is a financial incentive to help yourself when minor illnesses strike. Many a useful remedy is available for as little as 50p from the pharmacist and at the time of writing the prescription charge under the N.H.S. in Britain stands at £1.40 per item on the prescription. It is important to realise, however, that the chemist, or his assistant, does not know you as well as you know yourself. It is unlikely that you are going to give a full medical history when you go into his shop for your cold cure or for the occasional migraine or spot of skin trouble. It is unlikely, but quite possible, that you could buy, or borrow from a friend, something that is quite un-suitable for you and, as a result, instead of getting much better you actually get very much worse. This book has been written to stop this happening.

The second reason

A great deal of the information contained in this book refers, however, not to self-prescribed remedies and OTC medication, but to the medicines that doctors prescribe. Why is it necessary to include these in a guide to medicine? Does it mean that doctors are not doing their job properly and just handing over medicines without proper instructions—or warnings about possible side effects? There seems to be little evidence that the medical profession is, by default, letting its patients down in this way. There is, however, plenty of evidence to show that patients are often not really in possession of enough information to make their course of treatment completely safe or effective. This paradoxical situation: the concerned doctor and the uninformed patient has been created by several factors. Evidence shows that even if a consultation proceeds in the most ideal manner, with both patient and doctor having plenty of time to explain, ask questions and listen, less than 50 per cent of the information imparted by the doctor to his patient is remembered half an hour after the consultation took place. The reasons for this are legion and need not concern us overmuch here. Nevertheless this is a fact supported by carefully designed research carried out in several centres of medical excellence.

But if this is the case in conditions in which both patient and doctor are behaving 'ideally', what happens in other circumstances? For instance, in a clinic which is understaffed with, say, one doctor carrying the burden of work of his colleague as well as his own? Or if that doctor is himself less than efficient because of tiredness, lack of first class communication skills—or if he himself has a medical or social problem of his own? It is not possible to measure with any degree of accuracy how the patient's feelings at a consultation alter his, or her, ability to absorb or react to medical advice. Fear, somebody said, concentrates the mind wonderfully—but not on assimilating and retaining information—rather on 'fight or flight' activity. And we must never forget that for many good folk the results of all these investigations and tests add up to a very harrowing moment in their lives. In such circumstances getting out of the consultation room gains intellectual preference over listening carefully to instructions about how to take the drugs, what restrictions are to be observed and recognising trivial or serious side effects. No one has, to my knowledge, come up with hard facts on what measure of imparted information is retained by the patient when both the doctor and the patient are operating at low power on this score. A questionnaire might well put it at less than five per cent.

In the hospital context there should be a second, very valuable, method of information-sharing between doctors and their patients—the letter about the patient from the consultant or hospital doctor to the general practitioner. This, in theory, is in turn discussed with the patient. I doubt very much whether doctors or patients would wish, consciously, to be involved very much with an operation that only carried with it a five per cent chance of success. But still the appalling communication hiatus in medicine at present probably results in a five per cent transfer of information.

There are several good reasons given for this. Except in certain sections of private or professional practice the vital function of communication with the patient is often performed by junior doctors. The medical profession is a hierarchical structure the world over, and there is something of what, for the want of a better phrase, might be called a 'ladder of contempt'.

Almost all junior hospital doctors have a round contempt for the general practitioner or family physician whom they consider to be some sort of failed specialist who has 'fallen off the ladder' of medical (self) advancement. Of course as they slowly climb their own career ladder they learn better. But during these crucial years when they are often the main line of communication between the consultant and the G.P. and his patient they can do immense damage to the communications chain by filling discharge letters with masses of irrelevant detail and omitting the truly important treatment details.

Even when there is direct contact between consultant and general practitioner communications are often far from excellent. In many cases the consultant now feels somewhat uncomfortable in his task of imparting information to the doctor on the front line of medical practice. Becoming a specialist he has learned more and more about less and less of the whole gamut of medical practice. This being so, in the end (and that is in his heyday) he knows his own speciality very, very well, but very little of the broader principles of practice. So he will usually confine his advice to the family doctor very much to his own field. It is unlikely that he will stress side effects of the drugs he prescribes (even if he knows much more about them than anyone else). Neither will he dwell a great deal on drug interaction. He will assume that his colleague is well informed on these points and is often at pains not to talk down to the family doctor. Sometimes his faith is justified. In no case will he give more than an inkling of how much the patient has been told about his medication. This being so, the hurried or disinterested general practitioner assumes that his patient has been 'told everything' at the clinic or hospital, while very often the amount of information imparted to the patient in the busy clinic has been minimal.

This book is not attempting to create divisions in areas of practice for the medical profession and the pharmacist. The aim is to provide more knowledge about the medicines patients are taking—or, perhaps in the case of OTC medicines, the nature of the preparations they may be considering taking. In the interests of good medicine, doubts about a drug or remedy should always be clarified by discussion with the doctor or chemist. But to have (useful) doubts you need useful back-up knowledge. This is what this book provides.

How to use this book

Throughout the book, you will see the symbol ▲ set against certain medicines. This indicates that the preparation is available over-the-counter (OTC) at the chemist. It may *also* be available on prescription—when this is the case it will be indicated in the complete drug index at the back of the book. Prescription-only drugs have no symbol in the main body of the book, but will also be indicated in the index. The symbol (F) after a medicine indicates it is a National Formulary drug.

Every medicine dispensed by a chemist in this country has to bear its name. If it is dispensed from a hospital that name may well be typed on the label on the container. If you cannot read the name on your medicine, ask your chemist to print it so that you can. Every proprietary (OTC) medicine you buy has a trade name (and also bears a list of the ingredients). With the aid of these names you should be able to locate your medicine quite easily in the index at the end of the book.

Having located your medicine read the introduction to the section in which your medicine appears. Make sure that you are referring to the right section if this medicine appears in several sections. For instance, the same drug may appear in the chapter on Blood Pressure Remedies, and on Eye Medicines.

If it seems from what you have read that you should not be taking the medicine in question, or that you are experiencing adverse side effects, check with your doctor or pharmacist. It is important to remember that medicines are often complex substances that may act differently on different people. So, if you are worried check with your chemist or a doctor.

Most medicines work best if they are taken in the appropriate manner. Some should be taken with food, some before, some after meals. Some do not mix with 'social drugs' like alcohol or tobacco, others with certain items of everyday diet. Most important, many medicines do not mix safely or well with many *other* medicines. Unless you tell your doctor, or pharmacist, exactly what other medicines you are taking (including common everyday things like laxatives, the Pill or antacids) you cannot expect your doctor to know and warn you of possible problems. If in doubt read the 'Basic precautions' section on your medicine with particular care. If you appear to be taking a bad mix of medicines, consult your doctor or pharmacist.

Many people develop conditions like high blood pressure or glaucoma which involve a lifetime of medication. This affects them immediately in two special ways: if they continue their medication their illness is controlled, and their medical lifestyle is altered forever more. If you find yourself on long-term medication always check that any new medicine you take (on your own initiative or prescribed) suits you. That old friend that used to help you over colds or backache might not suit the new (medicated) you at all well. In fact, you could become seriously ill almost by misadventure. Using this book will help you to avoid this sort of unnecessary sickness.

Finally, four important aspects of medicine are not dealt with in *Good Housekeeping Guide to Medicines*. First of all, diabetes and its management are omitted. This is because most cases of the disease require treatment through injection, an involved procedure which is outside the scope of this book. At the same time, each diabetic is an unique case requiring the sort of intimate management that can only be properly carried out by a specialist in diabetes who liaises closely at all times with the diabetic patient.

Except in the case of the treatment of worms, medication for children is also omitted. There are also two main reasons for this. Firstly, many dosages for children are related to body weight and must be calculated by the doctor with special precision. Secondly, there are no N.H.S. charges on children's prescriptions and so medical advice can be readily sought and received by parents for all childhood illnesses—an admirable state of affairs which allows the primary care team to cater without any restrictions for the unique needs of children.

After much deliberation, it was decided to eliminate those drugs primarily concerned with the treatment of heart disease and blood pressure. This is because *all* the medicines used for management of such potentially serious problems *must* be obtained on a doctor's prescription, and are administered under strict medical guidance. The concerned physician will be most anxious to ensure that all his patients take their tablets correctly and safely. If you have any queries about such medication, *consult your doctor.*

Lastly, I have not dealt with the multitude of vitamin products on the market. The range is vast and ever-growing, and the pros and cons and ramifications of vitamin consumption would make a book in itself.

It is my hope that this book does something to dispel the mystique surrounding the doctor's office and the white coat of the chemist, and that the drugs you choose, or may be required to take, can be understood for what they are.

1

TREATMENT FOR PROBLEMS INVOLVING THE MOUTH, STOMACH AND BOWELS

Doctors talk about the gastrointestinal tract and the term is convenient medical shorthand for a system which starts with the mouth and ends at the anal canal (back passage). The system involves *digestion* (the breaking down of complex food-stuffs into less complex ones that can be absorbed by the body) and *absorption* of these nutrients and water into the body. Finally, *elimination* of (mostly) food waste products is effected through the lower bowels.

The word bowel has an innocent enough derivation, meaning a little sausage. But in our language it has taken upon itself something of a mysterious and dark implication. We speak, for instance, about the bowels of the earth. But when we consider medical problems involving the bowels it soon becomes evident that there is nothing very mysterious about these organs. Of course, their workings are 'internal' to some extent, but looked at in another way the contents of the gastrointestinal tract originate outside the body and, once consumed, usually manage their life-sustaining journey without conscious appreciation on our part.

The remedies in this section are primarily concerned with the problems of indigestion and over-activity or sluggishness of the bowels. Indigestion may be simple, or it may be complicated by ulceration. Certain areas of the gastrointestinal tract are prone to rather special malfunctions. For example the rectum develops piles and the anal canal may split and develop fissures.

An interesting but poorly understood factor in gastrointestinal disease is stress. The way in which stress produces symptoms in this complex system will be noted from time to time.

The mouth and gums

Digestion, of course, starts in the mouth where the saliva is mixed with the food and the breakdown of complex carbohydrates begins. The chewing of food (mastication) is essential for good digestion. This involves the teeth so good dentistry should meet with efficient health care. Unfortunately the professional expertise of doctor and dentist rarely work together and problems involved with the mouth and gums can become, therefore, a 'grey area' in which one profession usually assumes that the other is 'in control'. The patient lacks the benefit of either of their deliberations.

In this *Good Housekeeping Guide to Medicines* we will concentrate on the remedies for two common mouth problems, *gingivitis* and *mouth ulceration*. Fungus infections are dealt with in Chapter 7.

GINGIVITIS: CONDITION AND TREATMENT

This inflammation of the gums is often part and parcel of a more widespread disease: that of the crevice between the edge of the gum and its attachment to the neck of the tooth. This is sometimes referred to as pyorrhoea and should always be treated by a dental surgeon as poor oral hygiene, the deposition of calculus, and mal-occlusion secondary to irregular teeth, all of which prevent natural self-cleaning, are usually present. Because dental treatment often is rather expensive and delays in obtaining appointments are commonplace, remedies for local application are often indicated:

Remedies commonly used

SODIUM PERBORATE MONOHYDRATE AND HYDROGEN TARTRATE

▲ **Bocasan** (mouthwash)
- *Basic precautions:* Not advised in kidney disease.
- *Proper dosage:* Dissolve contents of sachet in 30 ml warm water. Use thrice daily as mouthwash after meals.
- *Side effects:* None.
- *Special advantages:* None.

CHLORHEXIDINE GLUCONATE

▲ **Corsodyl** (mouthwash)
- *Basic precautions:* If toothpaste is used before Corsodyl, rinse between applications. May discolour tongue and some dental fillings.
- *Proper dosage:* Rinse mouth for one minute with 10 ml twice daily. Course of one month suggested for bad cases.
- *Side effects:* May produce taste disturbances or skinning of inside of mouth and occasionally swollen glands.
- *Special advantages:* Inhibits *plaque* (calculus), useful after certain operations or in mentally or physically handicapped patients. [Also available as Dental Gel for brushing teeth.]

NIMORAZOLE

▲ **Naxogin** (tablets)
- *Basic precautions:* Not to be used by nursing mothers or by patients with diseases of nervous system.
- *Proper dosage:* One tablet twice daily for two days.
- *Side effects:* Mild nausea—may produce intolerance to alcohol.
- *Special advantages:* It inhibits the growth of certain (protozoal) organisms that complicate gingivitis problems.

HEXETIDINE

▲ **Oraldene** (mouthwash)
- *Basic precautions:* Do not swallow.

- *Proper use:* Rinse mouth with 15 ml thrice daily.
- *Side effects:* None other than mild local irritation.
- *Special advantages:* Safe and effective.

ACETARSOL

Pyorex (medicated toothpaste)

- *Basic precautions:* None.
- *Proper use:* Use as toothpaste twice daily.
- *Side effects:* None.
- *Special advantages:* None.

MOUTH ULCERS: CONDITION AND TREATMENT

Mouth ulcers occur for many reasons, some of which are quite mysterious. Factors that seem to influence the development of peptic ulcer (stress, injury) are implicated to some extent. Infection may play a part too. Some virus diseases of infancy are characterised by the appearance of mouth ulcers that heal, but which may reappear. Many people suffer from painful mouth ulcers from time to time; few escape them totally. Persistent mouth ulcers, however, may be a sign of gastrointestinal disease and a doctor should be consulted.

Remedies commonly used:

CARBENOXOLONE

▲ **Bioral** (a tube of gel)
- *Basic precautions:* None.
- *Proper use:* Apply thickly to ulcers after meals and at bedtime.
- *Side effects:* None.
- *Special advantages:* Sticks to mouth ulcer and promotes healing.

HYDROCORTISONE

Corlan (pellets)

- *Basic precautions:* Do not use if infection of the mouth appears obvious.
- *Proper use:* Dissolve in mouth as close to the ulcer as possible four times daily.
- *Side effects:* None.
- *Special advantages:* Lessens pain quickly and promotes rapid healing.

BENZOCAINE AND CETYLPYRIDIUM

▲ **Medilave** (gel)
- *Basic precautions:* Not suitable for young babies or for patients with sensitivity to local anaesthetics.
- *Proper use:* Apply four times daily to ulcer after meals.
- *Side effects:* None.
- *Special advantages:* Rapid pain relief.

CARBOXYMETHYLCELLULOSE

▲ **Orabase** (ointment)

WITH TRIAMCINOLONE

Adcortyl in Orabase

- *Basic precautions:* None.
- *Proper use:* Apply to ulcers after meals as required.

- *Side effects:* None.
- *Special advantages:* None. Adcortyl in Orabase offers rapid pain relief and speedy healing.

CLIOQUINOL AND VITAMIN C

▲ **Oralcer** (pellet)

- *Basic precautions:* Not suitable in cases of thyroid disease or for prolonged use.
- *Proper use:* On first day 6–8 pellets to be dissolved in mouth near to ulcer, reducing on second day to 4–6 pellets.
- *Side effects:* None.
- *Special advantages:* None.

ANTHRAQUINONE AND SALICYLIC ACID

▲ **Peralvex** (liquid)

- *Basic precautions:* Remove dentures. Not suitable in cases of salicylate sensitivity or if aspirin is being taken.
- *Proper use:* Paint on to ulcers four times daily.
- *Side effects:* None.
- *Special advantages:* None.

CHOLINE AND CETALKONIUM

▲ **Teejel** (gel), **Bonjela**

- *Basic precautions:* Not suitable in cases of salicylate sensitivity or if aspirin is being taken.
- *Proper use:* Using a clean finger massage in four-hourly.
- *Side effects:* None.
- *Special advantages:* None.

OTHER LOCAL ANAESTHETIC PRODUCTS

▲ **Rinstead Pastilles** contain menthol, myrrh chloroxylenol.

▲ **Rinstead Gel** also contains benzocaine.

▲ **Medijel** contains lignocaine and aminocaine.

▲ **Anbesol** contains lidocaine, chlorocresol and cetylpyridium.

- *Basic precautions, proper dosage etc.: See* benzocaine and cetylpyridium (Medilave).

The gullet (oesophagus) and the problems of hiatus hernia

The only real problems relating to the oesophagus are those of hiatus hernia. This is because the oesophagus is a transit organ: it conveys food from the mouth to the stomach. It therefore passes downwards through the chest and penetrates the large breathing muscle called the diaphragm. It is at this point—the gap or hiatus—where the gullet passes through the diaphragm that a hernia or displacement of tissues can occur. For various reasons (particularly obesity) the hiatus becomes enlarged and the normal valve-like function controlling the downward passage of food at this point breaks down. Whereas the normal person can stand on his head without his stomach contents 'refluxing' into his gullet, in the hiatus hernia patient the stomach contents tend to float up into the gullet from time to time even when he or she is upright. As the stomach contains acid this 'burns' the lower part of the gullet and produces the distressing symptoms of hiatus herniation. In the past, operation or restriction of activity (including sleeping in a semi-upright position) was the only therapy available for the hiatus hernia victim. Now modern medicine has much to offer, though the elevation of the bed still remains perhaps the single most important help that the patient can offer himself.

Remedies for hiatus hernia

ALGINATES AND ANTACIDS
▲ Gastrocote
- *Basic precautions:* May upset diabetic control because it contains sucrose (just over 1 g per tablet). Not suitable for patients on low salt diet.
- *Proper use:* 1–3 tablets chewed before swallowing four times daily after meals.
- *Side effects:* None.
- *Special advantages:* The alginates form a foam which holds antacids and coats the gullet. This neutralises the refluxed acid.

ALGINATES AND ANTACIDS
▲ Gaviscon
- *Basic precautions:* Granules and tablets contain sugar, hence unsuitable for diabetics; not suitable either for patients on low salt diet.
- *Proper use:* Suitable doses after meals four times daily (10–20 ml of liquid, 1–2 tablets chewed, 1 sachet).
- *Special advantages:* As for other alginate preparations—multi-preparation formulae allow for personal preferences in the manner in which preparation has to be taken.

ALGINATES AND CARBENOXOLONE AND ANTACIDS
Pyrogastrone
- *Basic precautions:* Not suitable for patients with heart or kidney failure or those on digitalis medication or similar drugs unless weekly blood tests vouch for its safety. Regular monitoring of blood pressure and weight advised.
- *Proper dosage:* 1 tablet chewed thrice daily after meals plus 2 tablets likewise at bedtime.
- *Side effects:* Fluid retention, hypertension, potassium loss.
- *Special advantages:* Carbenoxolone facilitates healing.

ALGINATES AND ANTACIDS
▲ Topal
- *Basic precautions, etc.:* As for Gastrocote.

Treatment of dyspepsia and peptic ulcers

(*See also* pages 22–25, Gastrointestinal spasm and its treatment.)

For reasons that are not very well understood, certain people suffer from symptoms (pain, discomfort) which seem to be related to a high level of acidity in the stomach. This may progress to pain on eating (often due to gastric ulceration) or 'hunger pain' occurring a few hours after eating (which may signify duodenal ulceration).

Today these two symptoms tend to be lumped together under the heading of *peptic ulceration*. The treatment of peptic ulceration is an important subject because, untreated, it can lead to complications of a life-threatening nature (perforation, haemorrhage, although this rarely happens today). The healing of peptic ulceration (in the proximity of the duodenum) can cause a stomach deformity associated with a delay, or obstruction, to stomach emptying. This condition (pyloric stenosis) usually needs surgical intervention. In the past, surgery also played a fairly large part in the treatment of peptic ulceration that did not respond to medical treatment. Nowadays, due to more sophisticated medication, this is less often necessary.

The mainstay of the treatment of dyspepsia, and peptic ulceration, involves taking substances that neutralise excess acid, or influence its secretion and promote healing. Although it would seem that factors other than excess acid in the stomach are involved in the incidence of peptic ulceration, the healing of peptic ulceration for practical purposes is largely brought about by the taking of alkalis which are provided in an almost bewildering variety by modern medicine.

A degree of consumer information on the score of antidyspeptic drugs may be provided under the categories of *simple* antacids and *compound* antacids. In addition there are *other* antacids which are best avoided and *antispasmodic remedies* that have rather specialised actions. Finally, a new category of specific *ulcer-healing drugs* has become part of everyday prescribing in recent times.

ANTACID REMEDIES

Simple antacid remedies

Active principal	Proprietary preparation	Formulary preparation
Aluminium hydroxide	▲ Alu-Cap	▲ Aluminium hydroxide mixture and tablets
	▲ Aludrox	
Aluminium phosphate	▲ Aluphos	
Magnesium preparations		▲ Magnesium trisilicate in various forms
Magnesium hydroxide	▲ Milk of Magnesia	
Sodium bicarbonate		▲ Sodium bicarbonate tablets

- *Basic precautions:* Patients on a salt restricted diet should not take sodium bicarbonate, and those with kidney problems should avoid magnesium preparations.
- *Proper dosage:* 1–2 tablets or 10 ml of liquid preparations taken when required.
- *Side effects:* Magnesium salts tend to cause loose motions.
- *Special advantages:* Bearing in mind the few restrictions, these are effective remedies for occasional dyspepsia.

Compound proprietary antacids

Generally, as the table below shows, the basic constituents of many of these compounds are similar. What is different is the presentation, the flavour and the care with which they are formulated.

Note: Dimethicone is an anti-foaming agent that is claimed to relieve flatulence.

Hydrotalcite is an aluminium/magnesium substance that is claimed not to be absorbed into the general system.

Pancreatin and pectin are claimed to cure dyspepsias caused by dietary imbalance.

Proprietary preparation	Alkaline ingredient	'Special' ingredient
▲ Actal	Aluminium and carbonate	
▲ Actonorm gel	Aluminium and magnesium	Dimethicone
▲ Altacite		Hydrotalcite
▲ Altacite plus		Hydrotalcite and dimethicone
▲ Andursil	Aluminium and magnesium	Dimethicone
▲ Antasil	Aluminium and magnesium	Dimethicone
▲ Asilone	Aluminium	Dimethicone
▲ Dijex	Aluminium and magnesium	
▲ Diloran	Aluminium and magnesium	Dimethicone
▲ Diovol	Aluminium and magnesium	Dimethicone
▲ Droxalin	Aluminium, sodium and magnesium	
▲ Gastalar	Aluminium and magnesium	
▲ Gelusil	Aluminium and magnesium	
▲ Maalox	Aluminium and magnesium	
▲ Maalox plus	Aluminium and magnesium	Dimethicone
▲ Phazyme		Dimethicone and pancreatin
▲ Polyalk	Aluminium	Dimethicone
▲ Polyalk suspension and gel	Aluminium and magnesium	Dimethicone
▲ Polycrol	Aluminium and magnesium	Dimethicone
▲ Prodexin	Aluminium and magnesium	
▲ Siloxyl	Aluminium	Dimethicone
▲ Siloxyl suspension	Aluminium and magnesium	Dimethicone
▲ Sovol	Aluminium and magnesium	Dimethicone
▲ Sylopal	Aluminium and magnesium	Pectin
▲ Bismag tablets and powder	Sodium and magnesium	

Antacids not generally prescribed by doctors

Ideas and prescribing practices in medicine are constantly changing. Accepted remedies quite often go out of favour with doctors while remaining firm favourites with patients. The following antacids are not often recommended by doctors for the following reasons:

Preparation	Reason
▲ Bisodol tablets	
▲ Calcium carbonate powder compound	
▲ Magnesium carbonate tablets compound	
▲ Magnesium carbonate powder compound	
▲ Maclean's tablets and powder	Contain calcium salts which may increase gastric
▲ Neutrolactis	acid, also cause constipation, high blood calcium
▲ Nulacin	and alkalosis
▲ Opas tablets and powder	
▲ Rennies tablets	
▲ Setlers tablets	
▲ Titralac	
▲ Bislumina	
▲ Lac bismuth	Contain bismuth which has been implicated in
▲ Moorlands tablets	central nervous system problems
▲ Roter	

ULCER-HEALING REMEDIES

Until comparatively recently the treatment of peptic ulcer was largely an amalgam of rest, release from stress, suitable diet, antacids and antispasmodics. (Peptic ulcer includes gastric ulcer and duodenal ulcer.)

Now a new generation of ulcer-healing agents are available. Perhaps the most interesting 'new' method of treating peptic ulcers has been the development of what are called H_2 receptor blocking agents.

Although the ultimate cause of peptic ulceration is shrouded in mystery and is probably multifactorial, the reason that once established ulcers sometimes do not heal is well known: the presence of gastric acid. This is why the use of antacids and surgery (removing the acid-secreting area of the stomach or interfering with the nerves that stimulate acid production) has been the mainstay of all ulcer treatment in the past.

Now it is possible to selectively 'block' the production of gastric acid. The secretion of gastric acid in the stomach is influenced by special cells called H_2 receptors. The H_2 receptor blocking agents effectively interfere with the function of these cells and gastric acid production falls considerably.

H_2 blocking agents

Active principal	Proprietary preparation
CIMETIDINE	**Tagamet**
RANITIDINE	**Zantac**

- *Basic precautions:* Malignancy must be excluded. Many doctors believe that positive evidence (visual) of ulceration, either as a result of X-ray or gastroscopy, is a prerequisite for the use of H_2 blocking agent therapy. *See* drug interaction chapter.

- *Proper dosage:* Cimetidine. Tagamet: 200 mg thrice daily with meals and 400 mg at bedtime. Sometimes in cases of duodenal ulcer 400 mg at breakfast and bedtime will suffice. Dosage may be increased, unless medically directed otherwise, if response is inadequate. Treatment should last for at least four weeks. Relapse may be prevented by a single dose of 400 mg at bedtime. As symptoms may be slow to settle in early stages of treatment an antacid may be combined with remedy until symptoms disappear.

  Ranitidine. Zantac: 150 mg twice daily for four weeks. 1 tablet nightly if recurrent ulceration is a problem.

- *Side effects:* Transient diarrhoea, dizziness, rash, tiredness are possible. Impotence and swelling of breasts has been reported in males. In elderly patients confusional states may occur. Ranitidine is claimed to have no serious side effects.

- *Special advantages:* May 'save' many patients from surgery. Reports suggest that up to 85% of ulcers heal with this remedy.

Other ulcer-healing remedies

CARBENOXOLONE
Biogastrone
1–2 tablets thrice daily after meals for 4–6 weeks.

Duogastrone
1–2 tablets thrice daily 20 minutes before meals for 4–6 weeks.

Pyrogastrone
1 tablet thrice daily chewed immediately after meals and 2 tablets at bedtime (has added alkaline and alginate).

- *Basic precautions:* Not suitable for very elderly patients or those with heart disease, high blood pressure, kidney or liver problems.
- *Proper dosage:* See above. Biogastrone is primarily recommended for gastric ulcer. Duogastrone for duodenal ulcer and Pyrogastrone for hiatus hernia.
- *Side effects:* If patients are liable to, or thought to be predisposed to water retention, disturbances of blood chemistry, cardiac or other problems, then routine weighing and blood pressure monitoring is necessary.
- *Special advantages:* These remedies are believed to promote healing by fortifying the intestinal cells against acid ulceration and by promoting the secretion of protective mucus. Young people are free from side effects and this makes these remedies an attractive alternative to cimetidine.

LIQUORICE
(also contains antacids)

▲ Caved-S, Rabro
- *Basic precautions:* None.
- *Proper dosage:* 2 tablets thrice daily lightly chewed and swallowed. For duodenal ulcer may be increased to 2 tablets six times daily.
- *Side effects:* Mild looseness of motions (rare).
- *Special advantages:* Is thought to act by increasing the number of protective mucus secreting cells, stimulating healing and reducing spasm. Some authorities are doubtful of its efficacy.

THE GASTROINTESTINAL SPASM AND ITS TREATMENT

The contents of the intestines are moved along by waves of contraction. This is an involuntary muscular activity and is called peristalsis. To produce peristalsis the muscular layers of the intestine contract and relax gently and involuntarily. Occasionally, however, instead of this smooth and gentle process the muscles go into a strong contraction. When this is sustained we speak of spasm, and spasm is often appreciated as pain of a 'colicky' nature. Sometimes the degree of spasm is slight—for example the 'hunger pains' we feel when a meal is anticipated, or the 'pain' that calls us to open the bowels. At other times the spasm can be acute, as in an acute attack of diarrhoea (*see* antidiarrhoeal remedies).

A group of medicines called *antispasmodics* are often prescribed as part of the treatment of peptic ulcer, the spastic bowel syndrome and diverticulitis.

There are several kinds of antispasmodic remedy. Some act directly on the muscle inside the intestine. Others dampen down on the whole of the bowel's natural function. These are called *anticholinergic drugs*.

Pharmacologists—perhaps more than other medical specialists—seem to love complicated 'shorthand' words that are baffling to the average person. To understand what 'anticholinergic' means it is necessary to explain the dual control system by which many of our automatic functions are regulated.

One arm of control is the sympathetic nervous system. This essentially prepares us to fight or flee. The pupil widens, the heart races, the muscles of our limbs tense and, as blood leaves our gastrointestinal system to be circulated to our organs of locomotion, digestion slows and the whole intestine develops a state of suspended animation. Once whatever has primed our sympathetic nervous system into a pitch of high activity passes, the second arm of our automatic nervous regulating system snaps into action. Blood is redistributed, digestion proceeds, the heart slows and the waves of peristalsis return.

Drugs that can produce sympathetic stimulation are adrenalin and its derivatives. The technical shorthand for these substances is to call them *sympathomimetic* (they mimic the sympathetic system). Drugs that produce parasympathetic stimulation are related to a substance called acetylcholine, and so drugs that produce parasympathetic stimulation are called *cholinergics*. Drugs that tend to 'knock out' or paralyse the parasympathetic system are called *anticholinergics*. If you think this is complicated and tortuous reasoning I will agree with you wholeheartedly. But it does define—and to some extent explain exactly—how certain drugs work and how they differ from other drugs that have similar effects, but act on different nervous pathways. This difference is particularly important with reference to side effects, as we shall see.

The direct action antispasmodics

Active principal	Proprietary preparation	Dosage
Alverine	▲ Spasmonal	1 tablet thrice daily before meals
Mebeverine	Colofac	

- *Side effects:* No special precautions or side effects are reported.
- *Special advantages:* Reduce spasm without side effects.

The strong anticholinergic antispasmodics

Active principal	Proprietary preparation	Formulary preparation	Dosage
Atropine	▲ Carbellon ▲ Neutradonna	Atropine sulphate ▲ Magnesium trisilicate and belladonna	0.25–2 mg daily
Hyoscyamine	Peptard Buscopan		Thrice daily

- *Basic precautions:* Not suitable for the elderly, in patients with glaucoma, in men with prostate problems, in heart disease. Not suitable in vomiting due to pyloric stenosis, for women while breastfeeding.
- *Proper dosage:* See chart.
- *Side effects:* Dry mouth, dilation of pupils with blurring of vision, sensitivity to light, flushing, dry skin, slow pulse, fast pulse, palpitation, difficulty passing urine and constipation. *Also see* drug interactions tables (page 193).
- *Special advantages:* These drugs have a powerful and quick effect.

The weak anticholinergic antispasmodics

Active principal	Proprietary preparation	Formulary preparation	Dosage
Dicyclomine	▲ Kolanticon ▲ Kolantyl ▲ Merbentyl ▲ Ovol		30–60 mg daily
Glycopyrronium	Robinul		1–4 mg thrice daily
Mepenzolate	Cantil		25–50 mg thrice daily
Pipenzolate	Piptal Piptalin		5 mg thrice daily
Piperidolate	▲ Dactil		50 mg 4 times a day
Poldine	Nacton		2–4 mg 6-hourly
Propantheline	Pro-Banthine	Propantheline tablets	15 mg thrice daily

- *Basic precautions:* Caution advised in patients with glaucoma, prostate or hiatus hernia as condition may be aggravated. Patients should not drive or operate machinery.
- *Proper dosage:* See chart. Usually best taken an hour before eating but see individual instructions.
- *Side effects:* Mild mouth dryness, thirst, dizziness, fatigue, blurred vision, constipation, poor appetite, dyspepsia. Headache and urinary tract problems are observed with some preparations, but on the whole these medicines are well tolerated.
- *Special advantages:* Tailored dosages to suit individual patients to reduce intestinal spasm and help with ulcer treatment. They also relieve the spasm-type pain associated with spastic colon or ulcerative colitis and in the management of colostomy cases.

The atypical antispasmodics

These antispasmodics are termed atypical because they do not act in the typical 'anticholinergic' way. They tend to increase the normal peristalic (propulsive) action of the stomach while stimulating the valve between the lower end of the gullet and the stomach to contract. This gently eases food along and prevents heartburn (caused by stomach contents 'refluxing' up the gullet) and also tends to prevent vomiting.

METOCLOPRAMIDE
Maxolon, Primperan

- *Basic precautions:* Not suitable for children or young adults unless under careful medical supervision as, very rarely, unpleasant side effects are reported. Not to be combined with atropine-type medicines.
- *Proper dosage:* Adults 10 mg thrice daily; dosage for young adults and children recommended by doctor.
- *Side effects:* Generally few, but in younger age groups there sometimes occurs a spasm of facial muscles and tongue, speech disturbances, eye rolling, and unnatural positioning of head and shoulders (*see* page 23).

● *Special advantages:* Can be prescribed in a variety of forms and they are very useful in diseases characterised by unpleasant or dangerous vomiting.

'Mixed bag' antispasmodics

The antispasmodic preparations listed below contain sedative compounds and others and their use is seldom recommended.

These preparations were largely introduced to 'try and persuade' difficult gastrointestinal problems to settle and thus save patients from surgery and from the complications of their illness. To what extent they succeeded is doubtful.

Nowadays, because surgery is safe and effective and new efficient ulcer-healing drugs are available, they should probably be allowed to slip into a limbo of half-forgotten cures. Many of these preparations contain barbiturates and sedatives which make them potentially dangerous and unpredictable in use, although doubtless many patients have benefited from them in the past.

▲ Actonorm (powder and tablets)

Contains aluminium hydroxide gel, atropine sulphate, calcium carbonate, diastase, light kaolin, magnesium carbonate, magnesium trisilicate, pancreatin, papaverine hydrochloride, phenobarbitone, thiamine hydrochloride.

▲ Actonorm-Sed

Contains dried aluminium hydroxide gel, belladonna tincture, activated dimethicone, magnesium hydroxide, phenobarbitone.

Aludrox-SA

Contains aluminium hydroxide mixture, ambutonium bromide, magnesium hydroxide, secbutobarbitone.

Aluhyde

Contains dried aluminium hydroxide gel, belladonna liquid extract, magnesium trisilicate.

APP consolidated

Contains aluminium hydroxide mixture, bismuth carbonate, calcium carbonate, homatropine methylbromide, magnesium carbonate, magnesium trisilicate, papaverine hydrochloride.

Bellocarb

Contains belladonna dry extract, magnesium carbonate, magnesium trisilicate.

Cantil with phenobarbitone

Contains mepenzolate bromide, phenobarbitone.

Libraxin

Contains chlordiazepoxide, clidinium bromide.

Pro-Banthine with Dartalan

Contains propantheline bromide, thiopropazate hydrochloride.

Stelabid
Contains isopropamide iodide, trifluoperazine hydrochloride.

Different kinds of diarrhoea

Diarrhoea may be caused by a dietary indiscretion or be due to food (or drink) poisoning. Food poisoning in turn may be due to the presence of a dysentery-type infection or may be the result of a toxin in the food. In the former case a specific antidysentery remedy in the form of an antibiotic may be necessary. If, however, a toxin is causing the problem such treatment will be ineffective and even harmful. Sometimes diarrhoea is due to a flu-like infection, so-called 'gastric-flu', in which remedies containing antibiotics may be possibly harmful because they tend to alter the normal flora and fauna of the gastrointestinal tract and thus cause fresh problems.

Chronic diarrhoeas are usually associated with structural changes in the gastro-intestinal tract and may be largely due to spasm. In the latter case the spastic bowel syndrome may be in evidence. The more serious chronic diarrhoeas of ulcerative colitis, Crohn's disease and diverticular disease all require special management.

Clearly, therefore, the management of diarrhoeas can be very simple, where a temporary condition of a non-threatening nature is involved and in which symptoms settle quite quickly, say in 24–48 hours. In effect the large majority of all attacks of diarrhoea are simple and rapidly respond to treatment. A subsection of these simple diarrhoeas are suffered by visitors to foreign climes and are graced with fancy names like *touristica, Montezuma's revenge* or even *Tokyo two-step*.

TREATMENT OF SIMPLE DIARRHOEAS

Remedies commonly used

CHALK AND KAOLIN PREPARATIONS

▲ **Kaopectate,** kaolin mixture (F), chalk powder (F)
There are no special precautions to be taken or side effects suffered. Dosages are arbitrary. A special advantage is absence of side effects and possibly a facility for absorption of toxins causing diarrhoea.

CODEINE AND MORPHINE/OPIUM PREPARATIONS

Aromatic chalk and opium powder (F)
Codeine phosphate (F)
▲ **Kaolin and morphine (F)**
- *Basic precautions:* Should not be used for patients of ulcerative colitis, spastic bowel syndrome and liver disease.
- *Proper dosage:* Codeine phosphate 45–120 mg daily in three to six divided doses. Kaolin and morphine mixture: 10 ml four-hourly. Aromatic chalk and opium powder: up to 5 g four-hourly.
- *Basic precautions:* In all diarrhoeas, especially those treated with sedative mixtures, at least 4–5 pints of fluids should be taken daily.
- *Side effects:* Occasional nausea, dizziness, sedation.

● *Special advantages:* Effective and economical antidiarrhoeal treatments that release the painful spasms of gastroenteritis.

DIPHENOXYLATE LOPERAMIDE
Lomotil, Imodium

● *Basic precautions:* Not suitable for children under one year, nursing mothers or for patients of ulcerative colitis and liver disease. May potentiate alcohol or sedative actions. *See* drug interaction table.
● *Proper dosage:* Diphenoxylate—4 tablets followed by 2 tablets four-hourly; reduce as symptoms clear (four 5 ml measures followed by two 5 ml measures of liquid are used). Loperamide—2 capsules followed by 1 capsule after each looseness of bowels.
● *Side effects:* Dryness of mouth (rarely), palpitations, sedation.
● *Special advantages:* Very effective with few problems if properly used.

DEXTROSE AND SODIUM CHLORIDE
▲ Dioralyte, Rehidrat

● *Basic precautions:* None.
● *Proper dosage:* 1–4 reconstituted sachets daily.
● *Side effects:* None.
● *Special advantages:* Replaces vital tissue fluids. Probably the best and safest diarrhoea remedy.

REMEDIES FOR OTHER DIARRHOEAS

Bulk preparations

Active principal	Proprietary preparation	Formulary preparation
Ceratonia	▲ Arobon	
Ispaghula	▲ Isogel	
Methylcellulose	▲ Celevac ▲ Cellucon ▲ Cologel	▲ Methylcellulose grans

Curiously, perhaps, bulk preparations (*see* Chapter 3, page 54) are often helpful in chronic diarrhoeas. There are no precautions involved. Dosage is arbitrary, side effects are negligible other than a tendency to experience colicky 'wind' pains especially at start of treatment.

Steroid preparations

Active principal	Proprietary preparation	Formulary preparation
Prednisolone	Codelcortone Codelsol Delta-Phoricol Deltacortril enteric Deltastab Precortisyl Sintisone	Prednisolone tablets

These powerful remedies are very much the concern of the physician in charge of the case. The precautions, side effects and special advantages are dealt with in Chapter 2 (see pages 45–48).

● *Proper doses:* In most cases an initial dose (of prednisolone) is 40 mg daily in single or divided doses until remission of symptoms occurs. Then dosage is reduced. Equivalent doses of proprietary steroids are given.

Anti-infective agents

SULPHASALAZINE
Salazopyrin

● *Basic precautions:* Not suitable if patient is allergic to salicylates, sulphonamides, methyl or propyl parabens or if other enema preparations are being used. Care needed if patient is on digitalis-type or foliate therapy, as drug tends to depress absorption of these substances. Blood checks should be carried out prior to and periodically during treatment.

● *Proper dosage:* (1) Plain tablets or EN tablets 2–4 four times daily—reduce when possible to 3–4 tablets daily and maintain indefinitely. (2) Suppositories—2 morning and 2 at night. Reduce after three weeks. May be used to supplement oral dosage. (3) Enema—1 enema at night.

● *Side effects:* Common—nausea, loss of appetite, raised temperature. Rare—anaemia and other blood problems, skin eruptions, painful joints, nettle rash, sore eyes, breathlessness, cough, mouth ulcers, headache, vertigo, tinnitus (ringing in ears), difficulty in walking, convulsions, insomnia, depression, hallucinations, infertility (temporary), urinary problems (urine may go orange).

● *Special advantages:* With such a formidable list of side effects, potential and actual, it might be thought that sulphasalazine offers no advantages. However, it controls most cases of ulcerative colitis and Crohn's disease effectively.

VANCOMYCIN
Vancocin

This antibiotic is used in potentially life-threatening situations. In such cases it is given intravenously and it produces several toxic side effects. When given orally it is not absorbed into the system from the gastrointestinal tract and can be useful in certain types of colitis. No special precautions need to be taken and there are no side effects when used in this way.

● *Proper dosage:* 1–2 g daily in divided doses.

Anti-allergic agent

Sodium cromoglycate is used extensively to alter the allergic response in asthma (see Chapter 2). A special preparation of the drug in gelatin capsules is used to inhibit the allergic response in diarrhoea caused by food allergy, in the treatment of ulcerative colitis and other bowel disease.

SODIUM CROMOGLYCATE
Nalcrom

● *Basic precautions:* None.

● *Proper dosage:* 2 capsules four times daily before meals. May be reduced, after therapeutic response, to the minimum dosage necessary to maintain freedom of symptoms. May be combined with other therapy.

- *Side effects:* Nausea, skin rashes and pains in joints occasionally.
- *Special advantages:* A remedy relatively free of side effects in an area in which such therapy is unusual.

POST-SURGERY TREATMENT

Surgery to remove diseased bowel can sometimes cause diarrhoea because of poor absorption of bile acids. The following drug helps to mop up these acids and settle the bowels.

Remedies commonly used

CHOLESTYRAMINE
Questran

- *Basic precautions:* Not suitable in cases of biliary obstruction. Any other medicines should be taken one hour before Questran.
- *Proper dosage:* 3–6 sachets daily, reducing in number if possible.
- *Side effects:* Constipation. Prolonged use may produce vitamin deficiency (A, D and K). supplementation with vitamins advised on long dose schedules.
- *Special advantages:* A useful aid to ileostomy and other surgery.

Remedies for constipation

Constipation can only be assessed in relative terms. This is very reasonable because a medical definition is almost impossible and 'sluggishness or inaction of the bowels' is as close a definition even a medical dictionary will dare. Bowel habits differ: some people will open their bowels three times a day, others three times a week, or even three times a month and find this state of affairs quite reasonable. They suffer no untoward symptoms, and this is their normal pattern of bowel action. In the past there has been an erroneous belief that frequent opening of the bowel is associated with a high degree of health. This has brought about a state of affairs that made people feel uneasy if their bowels did not move frequently enough, and so laxatives were taken routinely. For various rather complicated reasons that need not concern us here, the regular use of laxatives usually produces constipation, and some laxatives are worse than others in this respect.

There has been some radical rethinking with reference to the whole concept of laxatives over the last decade, and high fibre and bulk laxatives have taken the place of several 'old favourites' in the field.

Anyone considering taking a laxative should first examine the nature of the changes in bowel habit. Should a person gradually become more and more constipated relative to previous habits—or perhaps suddenly start to pass very frequent motions on a regular basis, then this *changed bowel habit* indicates the need for a visit to the doctor rather than the selection of a laxative.

Laxatives are grouped, for convenience, according to the way in which they act on the body. Thus we have: (1) Stimulating laxatives; (2) Bulk laxatives; (3) Laxatives that soften the motions; (4) 'Salts' type laxatives; (5) Suppository or enema laxatives; (6) Old-fashioned purging laxatives.

STIMULATING LAXATIVES

Remedies commonly used

BISACODYL

▲ Dulcodos, Dulcolax and Bisacodyl (F)

- *Basic precautions:* Do not crush or chew or take antacids within one hour of taking.
- *Proper dosage:* 2 tablets at night.
- *Side effects:* None.
- *Special advantages:* Produces soft well-formed motions without colic.

CASCARA

▲ Cascara tablets (F)

- *Basic precautions:* Not suitable for nursing mothers.
- *Proper dosage:* 1–2 tablets at bedtime.
- *Side effects:* Habituation. May colour urine red, colicky abdominal pains.
- *Special advantages:* None.

CASTOR OIL

▲ Castor Oil (F)

- *Basic precautions:* Not to be taken during pregnancy or menstruation.
- *Proper dosage:* 5–20 ml—taken on empty stomach.
- *Side effects:* Nausea, vomiting, colicky abdominal pains.
- *Special advantages:* None.

DANTHRON

▲ Dorbanex, Normacol, Normax

- *Basic precautions:* Not suitable for the incontinent or nursing mothers.
- *Proper dosage:* 1–2 tablets at night (Dorbanex), 1 tablet at night (Normacol), 1–3 (Normax) 2 × 5 ml granules breakfast.
- *Side effects:* Orange tint to urine, pink or red discolouration of anal skin, possible habituation.
- *Special advantages:* Efficient laxative.

FIG

▲ Califig, Syrup of Figs
(contains cascara, rhubarb and senna)

- *Basic precautions:* None.
- *Proper dosage:* 2.5–10 ml taken at night.
- *Side effects:* Habituation.
- *Special advantages:* An effective and safe laxative.

PHENOLPHTHALEIN

▲ Agarol and Petrolagar No. 2
(contains liquid paraffin)

▲ Bonamint, Brooklax, Ex-Lax and Sure-Shield Sur-Lax tablets
(all contain only phenolphthalein)

▲ Kaylene-OL with phenolphthalein
(also contains liquid paraffin)

▲ Nylax
(contains several ingredients including cascara, senna and aloin)

▲ Veracolate
(contains other ingredients)

▲ Phenolphthalein tablets (F) and Liquid paraffin with phenolphthalein (F)

- *Basic precautions:* It is possible that the laxative effect may continue for several days after a single dose.
- *Proper dosages:* Kaylene-OL and formulary tablets—50–200 mg at night; formulary mixture 5–20 ml; Agarol—5–15 ml; Petrolagar No. 2—10 ml; Veracolate—2 tablets at night; Bonamint—one chewing gum piece; Brooklax, Exlax, Nylax and Sure-Shield Sur-Lax tablets—one tablet.
- *Side effects:* Occasionally stomach cramps.
- *Special advantages:* Safe for occasional use.

SENNA
▲ Agiolax, Bidrolar, Senade, Senokot

- *Basic precautions:* None.
- *Proper dosages:* 1–2 heaped teaspoons with water before breakfast and after supper (Agiolax); 5–10 ml at night (Bidrolar); 5–10 ml at night (Senade); 2–4 tablets or 5–10 ml granules at night (Senokot).
- *Side effects:* Occasionally colicky pain; if this occurs reduce dosage.
- *Special advantages:* Extremely effective laxatives suitable for a wide range of patients.

BULK LAXATIVES

Remedies commonly used

Active principal	Proprietary preparation	Formulary preparation	Dosage per day
Bran	▲ Fybranta		6–12 tablets
		▲ Wheat bran	12–24 g
	▲ Proctofibe		4–12 tablets
	▲ Seven Seas Bran		1 sachet as needed
Ispaghula husk	▲ Fybogel		1 sachet twice daily
	▲ Isogel		2 tsp once or twice daily
	▲ Metamucil		5 ml 3 times daily
	▲ Vi-Siblin		10 ml daily
Methylcellulose	▲ Celevac		3–6 tablets or 5–10 ml granules daily
		▲ Methylcellulose granules	1.5–6 g daily
	▲ Cellucon		1–4 tablets chewed thrice daily
	▲ Cologel		5–15 ml daily
Sterculia	▲ Inolaxine		1–2 tsp daily
	▲ Normacol Antispasmodic		5 ml twice daily
	▲ Normacol Special		5 ml twice daily
	▲ Normacol Standard		5 ml twice daily
	▲ Normacol Standard sugar free		5 ml twice daily

- *Basic precautions:* These laxatives should be washed down with half a pint of water and plenty of fluids should be taken during treatment.
- *Proper dosage:* See table. Preferably taken after meals on a regular basis as treatment for constipation.
- *Side effects:* Some flatulence and abdominal distension is likely especially in the first week if these are being taken for diarrhoea, ileostomy or colostomy control. The side effects can be minimised by not drinking water half an hour before and after dose. Adequate intake of fluids throughout the day is mandatory.
- *Special advantages:* Bulk laxatives are Nature's cure for constipation. They also tend to help 're-educate' the bowel that has been misused by other laxatives and help in the management of certain chronic diarrhoeas and diverticular disease.

LAXATIVES THAT SOFTEN THE MOTIONS

These drugs act as mild laxatives, but also because they make the motion relatively soft and easy to pass they are useful in the management of haemorrhoids and anal fissure.

Remedies commonly used

DOCUSATE SODIUM

▲ Correctol, Dioctyl-Medo

- *Basic precautions:* Not to be taken in conjunction with liquid paraffin or anthraquinone derivatives.
- *Proper dosage:* Tablets range from 37.5 to 300 mg, to be taken two to three times daily with water (doses should start at high levels and gradually reduce as necessary). Elixir contains 12.5 mg of docusate per ml.
- *Side effects:* None.
- *Special advantages:* Safe and effective stool-softening laxatives.

LIQUID PARAFFIN

▲ Milpar, Petrolagar No. 1, Kaylene-OL and Liquid paraffin mixture (F), Liquid paraffin with magnesium hydroxide (F) and with phenolphthalein (F)

- *Basic precautions:* Not advised for prolonged use.
- *Proper dosage:* Up to 30 ml when required.
- *Side effects:* Leakage through anus, interference with absorption of fat and soluble vitamins; dangerous if accidentally inhaled.
- *Special advantages:* A cheap and effective stool-softener for short-term use.

'SALTS'-TYPE LAXATIVES

Traditionally 'a dose of salts' is thought of as a quick solution to the problem of constipation. Quite often it is. The 'salt' content of the laxative retains water in the bowel (by osmotic pressure) and this gives added bulk to the motions.

Remedies commonly used

LACTULOSE

▲ Duphalac, Gatinar and Lactulose elixir (F)

These are not 'salts' in the general sense, but act like them.

● *Basic precautions:* Not suitable for cases of galactosaemia (an inborn metabolic disease of children).

● *Proper dosages:* 15–30 ml of elixir in single or divided dose, reducing according to patient's needs.

● *Side effects:* Occasional colicky pains.

● *Special advantages:* Lactulose is virtually unabsorbed by the small bowel but is broken down in large bowel where it increases bulk of stool and stimulates evacuation.

MAGNESIUM COMPOUNDS

▲ Andrew's Liver Salts, Juno Juniper Salts, Magnesia, Epsom Salts, Glaubers Salts, Kest and Magnesium sulphate and hydroxide mixtures (F)

● *Basic precautions:* For occasional use; not suitable for elderly or for patients of kidney trouble.

● *Proper dosages:* Epsom salts, 1 teaspoonful in $\frac{1}{2}$ pint of water; the rest: 5–10 ml liquid preparation, 1–2 tablets, taken with water.

● *Side effects:* Some preparations cause excessive belching. Colic pains before defecation are common.

● *Special advantages:* Cheap, effective rapid-acting laxatives.

SUPPOSITORY OR ENEMA LAXATIVES

Remedies commonly used

Active principal	Proprietary preparation	Formulary preparation
Bisacodyl	▲ Dulcolax suppository	▲ Bisacodyl suppositories
Glycerol	▲ Practo-Clyss	▲ Glycerol suppositories
Phosphates	▲ Fletcher's Beogex	▲ Phosphates enema A+B
	▲ Phosphate enema	
	▲ Klyx	
Docusate	▲ Dioctyl-Medo	
Arachis oil	▲ Fletcher's Oil enema	
Magnesium sulphate	▲ Fletcher's Magnesium sulphate enema	
Sodium salts	▲ Micralax	
	▲ Relaxit	

These preparations are useful for treating stubborn occasional constipation. They also have the advantage of not entering the stomach and small bowel to produce the desired result. Enemas containing arachis oil or docusate and glycerol suppositories act by lubricating and softening the stools. *The majority of enemas come in single-dose disposable packs, and are best prescribed and used under medical supervision, at least initially.* For their side effects, precautions and advantages see under component drugs in the earlier laxative tables. The old-fashioned enemas (eg soap enemas) should be avoided.

OLD-FASHIONED PURGATIVE LAXATIVES

Remedies once commonly used, but generally now superseded

Active principal	Proprietary preparation	Formulary preparation
Rhubarb		Rhubarb mixture compound ▲ Rhubarb and soda mixture
Aloes	▲ Alophen Pills	
Mixtures of various purgatives	▲ Beecham's Pills ▲ Calsalettes ▲ Carter's Little Liver Pills ▲ Bile Beans	

Many proprietary preparations, and the few that remain in our formularies, are best avoided now that more modern and safe laxatives are available. The older versions very often have a drastic purgative action. Some have been shown to be capable, when taken in high dosages, of producing an abortion. Almost all are very habit-forming and produce more in the way of constipation than they can hope to alleviate.

Disorders of the colon and rectum

The intimate nature of bowel complaints often leads people to fight shy of going to the doctor. They will therefore tend to borrow or buy remedies to alleviate their distressing symptoms. With regard to the colon and rectum these could be soreness, discharge, and pain after the opening of the bowels. These are the result of piles, fissures or splits in the mucous membrane of the anus and when these are in the healing stage they will cause itching.

There is nothing intrinsically wrong with selecting one's own treatment for this kind of problem, provided the remedies are not being used improperly. If blood is being passed with the motions or is evident on the toilet paper, a doctor's advice must be sought. The same is true of conditions when an alteration of bowel habit becomes obvious. Otherwise a great deal of comfort can be gained from intelligent self-medication.

Medication for the rectum and lower bowel is considered under two sections: (1) Non-steroidal preparations; (2) Steroid preparations.

NON-STEROIDAL RECTAL AND ANAL SOOTHING PREPARATIONS

It is difficult to say exactly which constituent of a suppository or rectal ointment is really the active principal. In all likelihood it differs from patient to patient. One person may find that the pruritus (itching), soreness and excoriation often associated with piles or anal fissures are best treated by simple local hygiene, drying and powdering the anus. Others find that diet adjustments, the use of certain laxatives and so on (see page 32) are all that is necessary to ease their symptoms. The wide sale of OTC preparations is evidence that they are often effective. But more specific remedies are also sometimes called for.

(All preparations come in ointment and suppository form except *.)

Active principal	Proprietary preparation	Formulary preparation
Bismuth Hamamelis		▲ Bismuth subgallate compound suppository ▲ Hamamelis suppository ▲ Hamamelis and zinc suppository
Multiple	▲ Alcos-Anal ▲ Anodesyn. ▲ Anusol ▲ Germoloids ▲ Bismodyne ▲ Lasonil* ▲ Nestolyn* ▲ Preparation H *Ointment only	

- *Basic precautions:* Remember to remove wrapping on suppositories. Clean and dry external anal skin if ointment is to be applied.
- *Proper usage:* Suppositories—Insert 1 suppository into the bowel night and morning and after every bowel action. Ointment—Squeeze-fill applicator with ointment, insert applicator into anal canal and squeeze tube to introduce ointment into rectum and anal canal. To gauge the amount of ointment to be used experiment with tube and applicator before inserting applicator into the bowel. About twice as much ointment as the amount of toothpaste needed for teeth cleansing is adequate. Ointment may be massaged gently into tissues around the anus by finger covered with gauze. Length of treatment is a matter for debate. Though manufacturers may urge long-term use, physicians believe that if symptoms do not settle promptly medical advice should be obtained.
- *Side effects:* Some stinging or burning internally is to be expected. A sensitivity reaction to one of the multiple ingredients of proprietary preparations may occur in which case the physician must be consulted.
- *Special advantages:* Simple and effective ways of alleviating a very common problem. Piles may have been occasioned by mankind electing to walk upright and reducing the roughage intake necessary for easy bowel action.

STEROID PREPARATIONS—OINTMENTS, SUPPOSITORIES AND ENEMAS

Active principal	Proprietary preparation		Formulary preparation
Hydrocortisone	Colifoam Cortenema	enema enema	Hydrocortisone suppositories
Betamethasone	Betnovate Betnovate	rectal ointment compound suppository	
Prednisolone	Predenema Predsol	enema suppository	

Table continued on next page

Steroid preparations *continued*

Active principal	Proprietary preparation		Formulary preparation
Mixed steroid plus other ingredient remedies	Anacal	ointment	
		suppository	
	Anugesic-HC	cream and suppository	
	Anusol HC	cream, suppository	
	Hepacort Plus	cream, suppository	
	Proctofoam HC	foam	
	Proctosedyl	ointment	
		suppository	
	Scheriproct	ointment	
		suppository	
	Ultraproct	ointment	
		suppository	
	Xyloproct	ointment	
		suppository	

Qualities of ointments and suppositories

- *Basic precautions:* As for non-steroidal ointments and suppositories.
- *Proper usage:* There is always the possibility that important symptoms may be masked by the use of steroids. Close cooperation between doctor and patient is therefore very necessary. Some preparations favour the development of thrush. In such cases an anti-thrush antibiotic must be used simultaneously.
- *Side effects:* Few.
- *Special advantages:* The steroid soothing effects are predominant but these must be set against a high relapse rate on cessation of therapy.

Qualities of steroid enemas

- *Basic precautions:* Not suitable in cases with concurrent infection unless it is well contained by antibiotic.
- *Proper usage:* These are usually prescribed in single-dose disposable packs. The usual dosage is one enema administered at bedtime and retained within the body for at least one hour. Sometimes such an enema is retained more comfortably if it is warmed (by placing the complete bag in a bowl of hot water for a few minutes). The technique of use is for the patient to lie in bed on the left side 'curled up' with the knees drawn up close to the body. The stopper from the enema bag is then removed and the nozzle is lubricated with petroleum jelly or KY jelly and then gently inserted through the anus, which may also be lubricated. Once the nozzle is well introduced (about half of it will disappear) the bag should be gently rolled up expressing the contents into the rectum. This should be carried out as slowly as possible to make sure the enema is not rejected. With the bag fully rolled up the nozzle is withdrawn and the whole unit disposed of. For a few minutes the patient should lie face down and then any comfortable position may be assumed. Treatment is maintained for several weeks and then gradually reduced. Night-time use is recommended.
- *Side effects:* Long-term usage may cause general steroid side effects (*see* page 45).
- *Special advantages:* Steroid enemas will sometimes, by their local action, settle inflammation of ulcerative colitis and proctitis without creating the problems inherent in the oral use of steroids. The foam preparation Colifoam gives an enema-like alternative to patients who find enemas difficult to retain for long enough for their anti-inflammatory action to make itself felt.

TREATMENTS USED FOR PROBLEMS INVOLVING THE CHEST AND BREATHING

For the problems of infection see Chapter 4

Medicines and drugs can help with the management of diseases of the respiratory system in many ways. A simple simile to describe the function of the lungs is to look at them as a pair of bellows constantly pushing old (expired) air, heavy with carbon dioxide and light of oxygen, out of the chest and sucking in fresh air. This in turn re-oxygenates the tissues. If the lungs are not working efficiently enough the patient will quickly show signs of lack of oxygen—turning blue and becoming uncoordinated are among common symptoms. However, this simple analogy only reflects a partial picture of the problems of chest disease and disability. In addition to acute attacks, permanent or semi-permanent changes in the lung's structure also cause chest and breathing problems. Examples of this sort of occurrence include conditions such as pleurisy, pneumonia, bronchiectasis, lung abscess, lung cancer and so on. These are highly specialised medical diagnoses and not the sort of problem covered in this book. Treatment in such conditions is strictly medically controlled and patients are unlikely to be left with their prescriptions to make the best of things.

There is, however, a large number of chest problems of a recurring nature in which knowledge about the nature of medication can be helpful. While treating such problems, a prescription for a single or multiple drug is provided and quite often the chest patient is left pretty well to his own devices. In such situations OTC medications from the chemist will also play a part—often quite a large and important part. Some OTC medicines are particularly helpful in certain conditions, but many hinder recovery in others, especially if they are misused.

A concept of chest illness
A useful way to look at most chest illnesses is to imagine that the 'typical' ailment is made up of three components.

In the above diagram a chest problem is looked upon as a cake. The various components of the illness may then be viewed as very variable slices. Some chest problems—acute bronchitis, for example—will have a very large 'slice' of infection. The cake might then be divided as follows:

The allergy and stress factors are comparatively small and insubstantial. In asthma, the 'cake' is often sliced in different ways from time to time

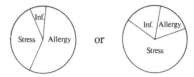

In other words, all chest illness is multifactorial. Often the blend of components changes with time and with environmental factors. The successful medical management of all chest disease involves helping the chest to react in a way that will counteract the various factors involved—in the knowledge that these will be multiple rather than single.

Remedies that help with wheezing

Wheezing of the chest, or *bronchospasm*, is a distressing, and medically important, symptom. It is possible to see quite clearly the working of the three-pronged activity of chest disease in bronchospasm. Often it needs two components of the 'cake' to set off an attack of asthma—say allergy plus infection or infection plus stress. The body may be able to resist one or other precipitating factor, but may not be able to cope with two and so the patient becomes ill. Fortunately over the last few years, particularly, many new and extremely potent remedies have been evolved that help to relieve this symptom by dilating (or widening) the smaller air-conducting tubes in the chest. These medicines are called *bronchodilators* and they work in various and rather differing ways. The information below details what may be expected in the way of response to treatment with assorted bronchodilators. If an individual fails to respond to inhaled bronchodilators, it may be a sign that additional therapy is required. The family GP should be consulted.

THE ACTION OF BRONCHODILATORS

The bronchodilators act in two different ways. One group of medicines is known as sympathetic stimulators (the technical term for these drugs is *sympathomimetics*, or *adrenoceptor stimulants*), and they affect the automatic (autonomic) nervous system which is a dual control system. One part of it, the *sympathetic system*, seems to prepare the body for 'fight or flight'. The heart quickens, the eyes' pupils dilate, the muscles tense and the air tubes in the chest widen—to allow for maximum air exchange on exertion. There is another part of the autonomic nervous system called the *parasympathetic*. This acts in a diametrically opposite way, 'closing down' breathing tubes, arteries and so on. In the treatment of bronchospasm, substances are also used that suppress the action of the parasympathetic system thus allowing the dilation and opening up of air passages in the chest. These are examined in the section on *anticholinergic treatment*.

The *sympathomimetics* are agents that *mimic* the sympathetic nervous system's action. They are used, therefore, to persuade the air passages in the chest to open wide—often in conditions in which one or more of the factors seen in the 'chest disease cake' concept are tending to make them contract and become smaller.

The sympathetic system can be stimulated in any of the following ways:

(1) Selectively stimulating certain cells in the air passages called beta$_2$ adrenoceptor cells.
(2) Generally stimulating the sympathetic system as a whole.
(3) Inactivating the parasympathetic system (thus giving the sympathetic system full reign to act).
(4) Using substances called Xanthines which relax the muscle fibres in the air transit passages and the coronary arteries and stimulate the breathing centre in the brain. (This is something of a high and infrequently realised therapeutic hope that may not, in fact, be realised.)

Not all bronchospasm is deemed to be asthma. In bronchitis, quite often, there is a degree of what would seem to be bronchospasm, inasmuch as that the chest sounds wheezy or 'musical' during breathing. This may be due to the presence of secretions in the air passages and to the resultant narrowing of important passages. The result is a 'noise' that the air makes as it passes through them (in the same way as a 'small-tube' instrument like a trumpet will sound different to a long-tubed tuba). The presence of infection does tend to trigger off real bronchospasm. This is yet another example of how the various factors in chest disease tend to aggravate one another.

Sympathetic stimulators—selective '*beta*' stimulants

Pressurised inhalers (aerosols) must be protected from sun and heat. Do not open or incinerate even when empty.

FENOTEROL

Berotec (aerosol)

- *Basic precautions:* It is claimed that there are no absolute contraindications to the use of this drug. However, in cases of thyroid, heart disease and high blood pressure the doctor must assess the case carefully. (Also *see* drug interaction chart.)
- *Proper usage:* Strict adherence to prescribed use is essential. 1–2 puffs inhaled from the pressurised measured dose inhaler may be increased to 2 puffs every four hours. If relief is not obtained the dose should not be exceeded and the doctor should be informed.
- *Side effects:* Temporary increase in heartbeat rate (palpitation), headache and tremor.
- *Special advantages:* A very safe and highly selective remedy (acting almost entirely

on the *beta* receptor cells in the chest). Its effect has a longer duration than many other similar drugs, thus reducing number of doses necessary.

ISOETHARINE

Bronchilator (aerosol contains isoetharine plus other compounds).

Numotac (tablets)

- *Basic precautions:* Not suitable for patients with thyroid problems, cardiac disease and high blood pressure.
- *Proper dosage:* 1–2 tablets, three to four times daily (starting with the lower dosage). Bronchilator: 1–2 inhalations, repeated after $\frac{1}{2}$ hour if necessary. Not more than 8 treatments in twenty-four hours.
- *Side effects:* Palpitation, tremor, giddiness.
- *Special advantages:* Highly selective action on *beta* receptor cells in chest. The tablet form of this drug is formulated with a special porous matrix (the material enclosing the grains of Numotac) to facilitate controlled and regular release of medicament.

RIMITEROL

Pulmadil (aerosol)

- *Basic precautions:* To be used with caution for patients with thyroid disease. Excessive usage of rimiterol may indicate lack of response and could place patient in jeopardy when urgent medical treatment or hospitalisation will become necessary.
- *Proper usage:* 1–3 puffs not to be repeated in less than thirty minutes. No more than 8 treatments in any twenty-four hours. The product may be prescribed in 'ordinary' or 'auto' form; the latter is a breath-actuated device with special instructions for use which should be strictly adhered to.
- *Side effects:* Feeling of anxiety, tremor, palpitation.
- *Special advantages:* A highly selective short-acting remedy (acting almost entirely on the *beta* cells in the chest). This is useful where relatively infrequent attacks of wheeziness need to be treated.

SALBUTAMOL

Ventolin

General note: The salbutamol medicines, marketed as Ventolin preparations, present a really effective spectrum of treatment for bronchospasm. The preparation comes in five forms for general use: (i) Inhaler; (ii) Rotacaps (an interesting inhalation substitute for patients incapable of using an inhaler); (iii) Spandets (long-acting tablets); (iv) tablets; (v) syrup.

- *Basic precautions:* Inhaler/Rotacaps—No special precautions except that caution is advised in use by patients of thyroid disease. Spandets/tablets/syrup—As above but these should not be combined with *beta*-blockers used for heart problems. If no relief from symptoms is obtained, seek medical advice promptly.
- *Proper usage:* Inhaler—Maximum 2 puffs, three to four times daily (1 puff before episodic, or expected, bronchospasm is often enough). Rotacaps—200–400 micrograms three or four times a day (one may be enough before episodic bronchospasm). The Rotacap has to be placed in a device called a Rotahaler which cuts capsule and delivers drug to chest during the breathing-in process. Spandets—1, night

and morning, swallowed whole and not chewed. Tablets—One 4 mg tablet three to four times a day. Syrup—10 ml of syrup three to four times a day. Lack of response to use of syrup needs urgent medical attention. Long-term use may increase dental decay, so routine dental hygiene necessary.

- *Side effects:* Inhaler/Rotacaps—None. Spandets/tablets/syrup—Fine tremor and occasional headaches and some dental decay for users of syrup.
- *Special advantages:* All the preparations are highly selective in their choice of *beta* receptors in the chest. This means that they work very well. The inhalation remedies are fast-acting and effective with smaller doses of salbutamol and so have fewer side effects. Spandets provide twice a day cover. Tablets and syrup can be used by patients who prefer to take medicines by mouth.

TERBUTALINE
Bricanyl
General note: Terbutaline preparations are marketed as *Bricanyl*. They are presented in four forms: (i) aerosol inhaler (auto/spacer and ordinary model); (ii) tablets; (iii) syrup; (iv) compound tablets and expectorant mixture.

- *Basic precautions:* To be used with caution for patients of thyroid disease. Do not combine with non-selective *beta*-blockers—*see* drug interaction table.
- *Proper usage:* Inhalers—1–2 puffs with a maximum of 8 puffs in twenty-four hours. Tablets and syrup—1 tablet or 10 ml syrup every eight hours. Slow-acting tablets—1 twice daily. Compound tablets and expectorant—2 tablets or 10–15 ml syrup at eight-hour intervals.
- *Side effects:* Tremor and palpitation.
- *Special advantages:* Specially effective as the preparations work selectively as chest *beta* stimulants. Compound tablets and expectorant contain sputum liquification elements and aid expectoration of mucus.

REPROTERAL
Bronchodil (aerosol and tablets)
- *Basic precautions:* As for salbutamol.
- *Proper dosage:* Tablets—20 mg thrice daily. Aerosol—1–2 puffs, three to four times daily.
- *Side effects:* As for salbutamol.
- *Special advantages:* As for salbutamol.

Other chest (non-selective) *beta* stimulants
Some remedies that were once popular are now being abandoned because they are less selective in their action as far as the chest is concerned. They tend to stimulate heart *beta* receptors and thus produce undesirable cardiac side effects.

ADRENALINE-TYPE
General note: These remedies contain adrenaline which is a potent dilator of air tubes in the chest. It also shrinks mucous membranes and acts as a cardiac stimulant. Physicians will sometimes give adrenaline by injection because it goes into action fast. In the past, remedies (based on a range of substances) such as

adrenaline and atropine spray, Brovon and Rybarvin inhalators were made for use with a small hand pump and these were very popular. Today, the Medihaler-Epi is used almost exclusively when adrenaline-like action is demanded, although some patients are dogmatic in their insistence that the old preparations work better. The roughly equivalent Medihaler-Epi contains adrenaline only, the Brovon pressurised inhaler and Brovon contain atropine as well (*see* next section) as does Rybarvin. This also contains other additives. For practicality they can be reviewed as a single group.

Medihaler-Epi
▲ Rybarvin, Brovon (pressurised inhaler)
Brovon (contains other ingredients)
Adrenaline and atropine spray (F)

- *Basic precautions:* Use with caution in cases of heart disease, high blood pressure and thyroid disease (*see* drug interaction table).
- *Proper usage:* Medihaler-Epi—1–3 puffs not to be repeated in less than thirty minutes; maximum 8 puffs in twenty-four hours. Brovon pressurised inhaler—1 puff every four to six hours; used to prevent acute wheezing—1–2 puffs not to be repeated in less than thirty minutes. Brovon—1–2 inhalations twice daily and once at night. Rybarvin—to be inhaled deeply for one to two minutes thrice daily. Adrenaline and Atropine spray—inhalations four times a day.
- *Side effects:* Anxiety, tremor, palpitation, dry mouth.

EPHEDRINE
Ephedrine hydrochloride tablets (F)
▲ C.A.M., Noradran and Ephedrine hydrochloride elixir (F)

General note: Ephedrine can be prescribed in tablet form, in which case it is the only ingredient. C.A.M. is a medicine in liquid form containing ephedrine and a substance called butethamate citrate. Noradran contains ephedrine together with other drugs.

- *Basic precautions:* The general safeguards relating to the use of adrenaline should be observed. Not safe for use in cases of prostate enlargement. Noradran is also a sedative.
- *Proper dosage:* Ephedrine—15–60 mg thrice daily. C.A.M.—20 ml four times daily. Noradran—10 ml four-hourly.
- *Side effects:* Tremor, palpitation, insomnia, retention of urine.

ISOPRENALINE
Aleudrin tablets, Iso-Autohaler, Iso-Brovon inhaler, Medihaler-Iso, Isoforte, Medihaler-Duo and Isoprenaline tablets (F)

General note: These are mainly isoprenaline-only remedies; Iso-Brovon contains added atropine and Medihaler-Duo added phenylephedrine. From the practical point of view they can all be considered together.

- *Basic precautions:* Use with caution in cases of heart disease, high blood pressure and thyroid disease.
- *Proper dosage:* Tablets—10–20 mg dissolved under tongue thrice daily. Iso-Autohaler and Medihaler—1–3 puffs not to be repeated in less than thirty minutes; maximum 8 treatments per twenty-four hours. Pressurised inhaler Iso-Brovon—1–2 puffs not more often than every thirty minutes. May be used four- to six-hourly as above to prevent attacks.

- *Side effects:* Tremor, palpitation.

METHOXYPHENAMINE
▲ Orthoxine
- *Basic precautions and side effects:* As for isoprenaline.
- *Proper dosage:* 50–100 mg every three to four hours.

ORCIPRENALINE
Alupent
- *Basic precautions and side effects:* As for isoprenaline.
- *Proper dosage:* Tablets—20 mg four times daily. Aerosol—1–2 puffs not to be repeated within twenty minutes. Not to be inhaled more than 6 times in twenty-four hours. Also available as syrup.

PSEUDOEPHEDRINE
▲ Sudafed
- *Basic precautions and side effects:* As for ephedrine.
- *Proper dosage:* Tablets—30–60 mg thrice daily. Elixir—10 ml thrice daily. Used more often for its effects on nose and sinuses than for chest problems.

Ephedrine-based asthma remedies
There are various OTC products popularly used in the treatment of asthma. Their actions and side effects depend on their composition.

Proprietary preparations	Composition	Dosage
Anestan	Ephedrine, theophylline salicylamide	1–2 tablets when necessary. Maximum 4 daily
Bronhipax	Extended action tablets. Ephedrine, theophylline, salicylamide	Maximum 2 tablets in twenty-four hours
Do Do asthma pill	Ephedrine, caffeine, theophylline. Most widely sold of this group for wheeziness, etc.	1 tablet thrice daily

The following prescription remedies are mixtures of various drugs. Their composition determines their side effects.

Proprietary preparations	Composition	Dosage
Amesec	Ephedrine, aminophylline	1 capsule thrice daily
Asmapax	Ephedrine, theophylline	1–2 tablets, thrice daily
Expansyl	Ephedrine, trifluoperazine, diphenylpyraline	1 capsule thrice daily
Franol	Ephedrine, theophylline, phenobarbitone	1 tablet, three to four times daily
Tedral	Ephedrine, theophylline	Suspension: 10 ml every four hours Tablets: 1 every four hours
Tedral S.A. Tablets		1 tablet morning and night

Anticholinergic treatments—affecting the parasympathetic system
These substances suppress the activities of the parasympathetic nervous system (*see* Chapter 1, page 23) and thus promote a sympathetic response. Such a response tends to dilate and open up the air passages in the chest. Such drugs have been used for treating asthma and the bronchospasm of bronchitis for years. Unfortunately side effects tend to limit their usefulness and because more helpful remedies are available they are much less used today.

IPRATROPIUM

Atrovent (inhaler)

● *Basic precautions:* Not suitable in the rare cases of sensitivity to atropine or for patients with glaucoma.
● *Proper usage:* 1–2 puffs three to four times daily—may be increased to 4 puffs. Unlike other inhaler-style preparations, its action is slow (thirty to sixty minutes) and so effectiveness should only be assessed after this latent period.
● *Special advantages:* May be more potent than the selective *beta* (chest) stimulants, especially in treating the wheezy, chronic bronchitic. Most anticholinergic remedies can be dangerous when used to treat persons suffering from glaucoma or retention of urine but ipratropium seems safe in such cases.

ATROPINE AND DEPTROPINE

Eumydrin, Silbe inhalant, Brontina, Brontisol and Atropine methonitrate and sulphate (F)
▲ Asma-Vydrin

● *Basic precautions:* Not suitable for patients with glaucoma and prostate disease.
● *Proper dosage:* Atropine/Eumydrin drops—For infants: 2–4 drops four-hourly, increasing according to manufacturer's instructions (*see* special advantages). Silbe/Asma-Vydrin inhalation—1–2 inhalations repeated after thirty minutes, maximum 12 inhalations in twenty-four hours. Brontina tablets—1 mg night and morning. Brontisol—1–3 inhalations every four to five hours; maximum 8 inhalations in twenty-four hours. Also contains isoprenaline. Basic precautions as for isoprenaline.
● *Side effects:* Dry mouth, blurred vision, difficulty in passing urine.
● *Special advantages:* Eumydrin is particularly useful in the bronchospasm of whooping cough. Brontina, Brontisol useful if excess secretion in chest complicates wheeziness—especially chronic bronchitis. Silbe, Asma-Vydrin also contain adrenalin.

Xanthine bronchodilators
These drugs may occasionally produce the needed dilation of the air tubes in the chest when other remedies fail. Unfortunately the side effects (nausea, headache) may be severe but these have been modified in newer sustained-release (slow-release) compounds. Xanthine compounds are widely used in combination with other drugs and this makes for difficult analysis of their side effects or special advantages. In order to use Xanthines to the best advantage, medicines are manufactured in several forms, especially as suppositories to prevent gastric upsets. Xanthine chemicals have names that end in *phylline* or *fylline*. To understand the bewildering variety of these compounds the following table may be consulted.

Compound of Xanthine	Proprietary and formulary preparations	Type O = oral R = rectal	Dosage
Acepifyllines	▲ Etophylate	O R	3 g per day 1.5 g per day
Aminophyllines	▲ Aminophylline (F)	O R	100–300 mg per day 360 mg once or twice daily
	▲ Cardophylin	O	100–300 mg per day
	▲ Phyllocontin	O	225 mg twice daily (swallowed whole)
	▲ Theodrox	O	195 mg thrice daily
	▲ Theo-dur	O	300–450 mg per day
Theophyllinate	▲ Choledyl	O	100–400 mg four times per day
Diprophylline	▲ Silbephylline	O & R	200 mg tablet one to two times daily or suppositories, 1 every twelve hours
Etamiphylline	Millophyline	O & R	100 mg three to four times daily or 1–2 suppositories daily
Proxyphylline	▲ Thean	O & R	1 tablet three times daily plus 1 suppository at night
Theophylline	▲ Theophylline (F)	O	60–200 mg three to four times per day
	▲ Monotheamin	O	400–800 mg per day
	▲ Nuelin	O	1–2 tablets thrice daily
	▲ Nuelin SA	O	1 tablet twice daily
	▲ Rona-Slophyllin	O	250–500 mg twice daily
	▲ Theocontin Continuus	O	200 mg twice daily
	▲ Theograd	O	2 tablets initially, followed by 1 tablet twelve-hourly

- *Basic precautions:* Not suitable in liver disease, epilepsy or during lactation.
- *Proper dosage:* According to manufacturer's dosage instructions (*see* above).
- *Side effects:* Palpitation, nausea, heart irregularity, soreness if given rectally for prolonged periods.
- *Special advantages: See* earlier general paragraph.

THE USE OF STEROIDS

The general automatic function of the body is a complex process and is in part mediated by the activity of several glands. These secrete various special chemical substances into the bloodstream. This allows for a very sensitive control of various tissues and organs in the body. The glands are called endocrine glands and the chemicals they produce hormones. Two glands, situated over the kidneys, and thus called adrenals, are implicated in producing a group of hormones, the adreno-cortical hormones (so called because they come from the outside, or cortex, of the glands). One group of these hormones is called glucocorticoids (because one of their functions is involved in action upon blood glucose). Our interest however is mainly in another attribute of these glucocorticoids—their ability to reduce inflammatory changes and certain allergic and rheumatic processes in the body. To start with these 'wonder drugs' were called corticosteroids (because chemically they belong to a group of substances referred to as steroids and also because they come from the cortex of the gland in question). Now we just say steroids and the term has been applied to not only the actual hormones produced by the adrenal gland but to a large number of synthetic substances which act like the natural substance produced in the adrenals.

It is perhaps paradoxical that the therapeutic use of steroids discussed in this book is in a way quite unrelated to their *natural* function. Thus, when a steroid is prescribed as an anti-inflammation or anti-allergy remedy, in many cases its *natural* function within the body is reflected in the side effects that the particular drug produces.

It is important to remember too that, in some cases, one function of a steroid that is being actively courted for treatment (one might for example be using it for its potent antiallergic function) may cause problems because it also has an anti-inflammation function (and thus stops the body reacting with its normal defence measures to infection).

Physicians always, quite rightly, look upon steroids as potent and potentially dangerous drugs, particularly because they work so magically and dramatically in certain situations. They are often abused by patients, with subsequent long-term harmful effects. They are therefore always administered as prescription drugs.

Steroid medication can damp down or even totally suppress natural steroid function. Very careful and gradual withdrawal of steroid therapy is necessary when treatment is terminated. Nevertheless, steroids have an important part to play in the treatment of many diseases—especially chest diseases.

Steroids can be life-saving agents when administered by injection in acute conditions of asthma. But this aspect does not really concern this book. There are two ways in which steroids can be used in the context of home management and which we will discuss: (i) inhalers containing steroids; (ii) steroids in tablet form.

Steroid inhalers

Nobody knows exactly how steroids relieve spasm of the bronchial tubes, but there is no doubt that they work extremely well. Because much smaller doses of steroids can be effective in this form, troublesome side effects can be kept to a minimum. If there is too great a degree of spasm present, or too much mucus in the airways to allow the steroid to reach the cells of the air tubes, then sometimes a broncho-dilator aerosol can be used before the steroid aerosol is used.

Or the problem may be relieved in another way. If the chest condition is complicated by infection this can be relieved by antibiotics.

BECLOMETHASONE AND BETAMETHASONE

These two steroids are used in inhalation therapy. The two derivative proprietary preparations are

Becotide and Bextasol

Becotide is produced in two forms—as an inhaler and in the form of insufflation cartridges called Rotacaps which are manufactured in two strengths. The Rotacaps are used in a small device called Rotahaler. Bextasol is an aerosol inhaler.

● *Basic precautions:* Not suitable for patients with tuberculosis.

● *Proper usage:* It is important to stress that Becotide and Bextasol should be thought of as a regular medication, not as a remedy for acute attacks of wheezing, although they occasionally have this effect. The usual dose for the aerosol is 2 puffs three or four times daily; for Rotacaps it is 200 micrograms three or four times daily.

- *Side effects:* Thrush (candidiasis), which is a fungus infection of the mouth, occasionally occurs. This usually responds to suitable treatment (*see* Fungal infections, pages 67–70 and 83). Hoarseness may also occur.
- *Special advantages:* Produces the beneficial subjective effects of steroid therapy with little in the way of steroid side effects. May be used to aid the transfer, for patients on oral steroids, to safer inhalation therapy.

Steroid tablets

A large number of steroid tablets are in use and a bewildering number of compounds are marketed. Medical supervision is always mandatory. Sometimes, because of discontinuance or unavailability of local supply, changes in type or brand of steroid may be necessary. The chart below helps in the calculation of equivalent dosages. The doses given are for anti-inflammatory action. But anti-allergic dosage is similar. Prednisolone is the most common steroid taken by mouth and so heads the list.

Active principal	Equivalent dose of proprietary preparation		Tablet sizes of formulary preparations		Dosage per day
Prednisolone	Codelcortone	5 mg	Prednisolone	1–5 mg	Up to 30 mg
	Delta-Phoricol	5 mg			
	Deltacortril Enteric	2.5 and 5 mg			
	Deltastab	1 and 5 mg			
	Precortisyl	1 and 5 mg			
	Prednesol	5 mg			
	Sintisone	6.65 mg			
Prednisone (body converts this to prednisolone)	Decortisyl	1 and 5 mg	Prednisone	1 and 5 mg	Up to 30 mg
	Deltacortone	5 mg			
Betamethasone	Betnelan	500 micrograms			Up to 5 mg
	Betnesol	500 micrograms			
Dexamethasone	Decadron	500 micrograms			Up to 3 mg
	Dexacortisyl	500 micrograms			
	Oradexon	500 micrograms			
Hydrocortisone	Hydrocortistab	20 mg			Up to 30 mg
	Hydrocortone	10 mg			
Methylprednisolone	Medrone	2 and 4 mg			Up to 16 mg
Paramethasone	Metilar	2 mg			Up to 8 mg
Triamcinolone	Adcortyl	1 and 4 mg	Triamcinolone	4 mg	Up to 24 mg
	Ledercort	2 mg			

General note: The use of these steroid tablets is subject to basic stipulations, listed below.

- *Basic precautions:* Not suitable for patients with tuberculosis, herpes, peptic ulcer, certain kidney diseases, myasthenia, osteoporosis (brittle bones), recent surgery, diverticulitis, thrombophlebitis (deep vein thrombosis), psychological disturbances, pregnancy, local or other infections.

- *Proper dosage:* Doctors' instructions must be observed strictly. Generally speaking, dosage is adjusted to the lowest possible in order to obviate symptoms. Some steroids are given on special short-term courses.
- *Side effects:* Because steroids suppress symptoms of infection, it is imperative for patients to be seen by a doctor even if they have relatively minor symptoms. Some side effects include a moon face (a curious blown-up bland, rather expressionless face), striae (stretch marks), acne, buffalo hump (a deformity of the neck), osteoporosis, stoppage of periods, mental upset, thrombosis disorders, peptic ulceration, bleeding from gastrointestinal tract, headache, insomnia, fatigue, rashes, excess hair growth, dizziness, cataracts, pancreatitis, lack of appetite.
- *Special advantages:* Although steroid therapy is fraught with danger, especially if not carefully and responsibly managed, it can be life-saving in a wide variety of illness that cannot otherwise be controlled. Steroid therapy is a powerful agent to be reserved for dangerous diseases.

Prevention of asthma

There are many ways of preventing asthma and in this context the 'slice of cake' analysis of chest problems generally (*see* pages 37–38) is particularly pertinent. Reducing stress, allergy or infection always pays certain dividends in the management of asthma and wheeziness.

The reduction of any allergic component in asthma is always an attractive option. The prevention of the presence of allergic stimuli, wherever possible, always adds to the freedom from attacks and has led to various suggestions on the management of asthma. Some of these relate to dust-free surroundings, plant-free environments, the elimination of certain pets whose dander may be a stimulus to asthma, even dietary modifications (the 'Stone Age' diet). These, when adhered to by some people, have led to a striking reduction in wheeziness. Desensitisation procedures have also made a remarkable improvement in the case of certain patients, but are outside the scope of this book.

Relatively new ways have been discovered to influence, by medicines, these cells which seem to liberate the chemical mediators in asthma and wheeziness. Although the wide range of drugs called *antihistamines* are useful in the management of certain types of allergy (i.e. hay fever and some skin allergies, *see* pages 148 and 87), they have little or no effect in asthma proper. Happily, a drug has been developed which has been shown to be particularly useful in the prevention of asthma.

This new drug seems to act by *stabilising* the activity of certain cells in the body (called mast cells) which are (abnormally) involved in the liberation of various mediator substances. Once these substances enter the circulation, in appreciable amounts, they trigger off the wheezy asthmatic response in the chest's air-conducting tubes. It is possible too that these stabilising substances may also act to dampen down the receptor cells in the air tubes which are involved in producing unwanted bronchospasm.

SODIUM CROMOGLYCATE

Intal, Intal Co (contains added isoprenaline)

- *Basic precautions:* It is essential to remember that these remedies have no place in the *treatment* of asthma or wheeziness. For this other remedies are necessary. Cromoglycate prevents attacks of asthma which may be due to allergy, exercise, cold air or chemical or occupational irritants. The drug has to be taken regularly and inhaled in the form of *spincaps* from a special plastic *spinhaler* or as *Intal Nebuliser Solution* from a power-operated nebuliser. Also *Intal* (metered dose aerosol) *Inhaler*—2 puffs four times daily or before any activity likely to produce wheezing. There are no contraindications to treatment.

- *Proper dosage:* The normal dose is 1 spincap inhaled four times a day. A satisfactory routine is for 1 to be taken in the morning and at night and at intervals of three to six hours during the day. It is safe to increase this to eight times a day if exposure to known 'trigger' factors is anticipated or feared. Once the asthmatic state has become stabilised and attacks are diminished, then dosage may be gradually reduced. If it is decided to discontinue prophylaxis this should be done gradually over at least a week.

- *Side effects:* Occasional irritation to the throat and upper air passages may occur. The manufacturers suggest that this is an indication for the substitution of Intal Co for plain Intal. Others would stress that a bronchodilator aerosol should be used just before Intal inhalation. In practice both procedures seem to work satisfactorily. It is very rarely that the irritation to the powdered cromoglycate makes it necessary to abandon treatment.

- *Special advantages:* The prevention of asthma allows freedom from the many drug regimes associated with the management of this common and unpleasant condition. Intal, in many cases, also allows for a reduction or elimination of steroid therapy administered in more severe types of asthma. Slow rates of reduction of steroids are mandatory in such cases and a doctor must supervise the whole operation. The frequency of other bronchodilator remedies can also be affected with cromoglycate therapy.

Cough mixtures

Doctors, when they are learning their art, are often reminded that there is no real advantage in being the first to try a new remedy or in being the last physician to discard the old one. This is good advice. There is a fashionable tendency in modern prescribing to write off many well-tried and useful remedies in the name of science. The *British National Formulary*, a reputable guide to prescribing, published jointly by the British Medical Association and the Pharmaceutical Society of Great Britain, has had some hard words to say about cough mixtures in general—particularly expectorant cough mixtures (taken to help shift mucus from the chest). It stresses that there is no scientific basis for prescribing such cough mixtures, despite the fact that millions of patients seek and find both doctors' and OTC remedies on this score very definitely helpful. The reason for this curious discrepancy seems inexplicable.

From a more practical point of view, one should look at the function of cough medicines. There are those that make it easier to cough up sputum from the chest (the expectorants) and those that tend to prevent coughing (broadly speaking, the linctuses). Sometimes, because of local irritation of the tissues, the chest responds excessively to the stimulus of quite small quantities of mucus. This is an irritating but 'useless' cough that the linctus helps to soothe.

THE SELECTION OF COUGH MEDICINES

Many cough mixtures reflect the medical beliefs and principles of a bygone age when poly-pharmacy ruled supreme and unless a mixture contained at least half a dozen or so ingredients it was judged to be inelegant and ineffective. The modern trend is to concentrate on simple medicines, perhaps containing but one ingredient. Such preparations possibly lack finesse and, not unimportantly, flavour too. Generally speaking, those who seek a suitable cough mixture should pick one with the fewer rather than the greater number of ingredients, especially if other drugs are being taken at the same time.

Examples of stimulating cough medicines (expectorants)

Proprietary or formulary preparation	Components and comments
▲ Actifed Expectorant	Contains pseudoephedrine an antihistamine and guaiphenesin.
▲ Ammonium Chloride Mixture (F) ▲ Ammonium and Ipecacuanha Mixture (F) ▲ Ammonium Chloride and Morphine Mixture (F) ▲ Ipecacuanha and Morphine Mixture (F)	All traditional cough mixtures. Those containing morphine (in small doses) are warming and popular with sufferers of chronic bronchitis. Few side effects.
Alupent Expectorant	Contains a bronchodilator and substance that liquifies mucus. Occasional side effects: palpitation, headache, nausea. Not suitable for patients with thyroid disease.
▲ Benylin Expectorant	Contains an antihistamine. May cause drowsiness. Avoid alcohol, driving or operating machinery. A well-tried and safe expectorant.
Bronchotone	Contains several drugs which may cause side effects: ephedrine, salicylates, caffeine, iodine and belladonna. Side effects as for individual components.
▲ Dimotane Expectorant	A complex formulation. Not suitable for epileptics or brain-damaged patients, or for those with glaucoma, thyroid or heart disease. Not to be taken in conjunction with many other drugs. Best used as a prescribed product.
▲ Famel Expectorant	Contains guaiphenesin.
▲ Franol Expectorant	Contains a barbiturate and other compounds.
Franolyn Expectorant	Contains ephedrine and theophylline.
▲ Galloways Bronchial Expectorant	Contains squill, ipecacuanha, aniseed and chloroform.
▲ Phenergan Compound Expectorant	Contains an antihistamine. A well-tried and safe expectorant.
▲ Pholcomed Expectorant Syrup	Contains guaiphenesin and methyl ephedrine.
▲ Pulmo Bailly	Contains guaicol and codeine.

Proprietary or formulary preparation	Components and comments
▲ Sudafed Expectorant	Contains pseudoephedrine. Should be used with care in heart disease, diabetes. *See* drug interaction table.
Tedral Expectorant	Contains ephedrine, diprophylline and guaiphenesin.
▲ Tussifans Mixture	An old-fashioned yet safe expectorant.
Vallex	'Mixed' expectorant; may cause drowsiness and confusion.
▲ Vicks Expectorant Cough Syrup	Contains guaiphenesin.

Sedative cough medicines (linctuses)

Proprietary or formulary preparation	Components and comments
▲ Antussin	Dextromethorphan, ammonium chloride, ipecacuanha.
Benylin with Codeine	Antihistamine action of benadryl, plus codeine. (It is actually also OTC, but most chemists do not sell because of abuse.)
▲ Benylin Fortified	Dextromethorphan and sodium citrate. Acts to suppress 'dry' cough.
▲ Codeine Linctus (F) ▲ Pholcodine Linctus ▲ Diatuss	Simple linctus preparations suitable for occasional use; especially at night to prevent sleep being disturbed by coughing. (Many chemists do not sell Codeine Linctus because of abuse.)
▲ Cosylan	Dextromethorphan.
▲ Covonia	Dextromethorphan, guaiphenesin menthol.
Diamorphine Linctus (F)	This is a powerful linctus which is reserved usually for the treatment of intractable coughing, under strict medical supervision.
▲ Famel Original	Creosote, codeine.
▲ Famel Linctus	Pholcodine, papaverine.
▲ Galloways Cough Syrup	Ipecacuanha, squill, acetic acid, chloroform, ether.
▲ Hills Bronchial Balsam	Ammonium acetate, capsicum, benzoin, ipecacuanha, morphine. To be used by adults only.
▲ Hills Junior Balsam	Benzoin, ipecacuanha, lobelia, capsicum, ammonium acetate.
▲ Liqufruta	Garlic, aniseed, linseed, peppermint, liquorice, ipecacuanha.
▲ Owbridges Cough Syrup	Cetylpyridinium bromide, ammonium acetate, clove, aniseed, capsicum.
Phensedyl Linctus	Seldom sold OTC due to drug abuse.
Pholcolix	Pholcodine, paracetamol and phenylpropanolamine. To be used for coughs with common cold, but though it is also OTC, it is best regarded as a prescribed product.
▲ Pholcomed and Pholcomed Forte and Pholcomed Pastilles ▲ Pholcomed Diabetic and Pholcomed Forte Diabetic	Pholcodine presented in an ion-exchange resin form. In this form the drug is normally needed only twice daily. The two diabetic preparations contain no sugar.

Table continued on next page

Sedative cough medicines (linctuses) (*continued*)

Proprietary or formulary preparation	Components and comments
▲ Squill Linctus Opiate (F) Dimyril Linctus ▲ Sancos ▲ Benafed ▲ Actifed Compound Linctus ▲ Copholco ▲ Davenol ▲ Extil Compound ▲ Lotussin ▲ Tixylix Valledrine	These are multi-formulation remedies and are liable to produce the side effects of their combined contents. In practice, however, because they are only used occasionally and at night, side effects are few and quite acceptable.
▲ Tancolin	Theophylline and dextromethorphan. To be used for children.
▲ Venos Original	Glucose, molasses, capsicum, aniseed and camphor.
▲ Venos Honey and Lemon	Lemon, honey, ammonium chloride and ipecacuanha.
▲ Venos Adult Formula	Contains noscapine.
▲ Vicks Formula 44	Sodium citrate, dextromethorphan, cetylpyridinium.
▲ Vicks Cough Calmers	Boiled sweet lozenge containing dextromethorphan and benzocaine.

Other cough medicines

Yet another kind of cough medicine is the *elixir*. This is regarded as a general purpose remedy which may be helpful when coughing becomes a problem. There are some simple formulations such as those detailed below.

LINCTUS ELIXIR REMEDIES

▲ Robitussin and Organidin

These drugs are preferable to mixtures like *Dimotane Expectorant*, *Exyphen*, *Linctifed Expectorant* and *Triominic Elixir*, where the formulation is more complicated. Since elixir-type cough remedies tend to be taken more frequently than linctuses, however, side effects can be more of a problem.

MUCOLYTIC REMEDIES

Bisolvon, Mucolex, Mucodyne

A fairly recent addition to cough mixtures generally has been the introduction of medicines called *mucolytics*. *Bisolvon*, *Mucolex* and *Mucodyne* are examples of these. They are all prescription-only medicines and are thought to reduce the stickiness of bronchial secretions; side effects are rare and there seem to be no special precautions involved in their use.

▲ Cough mixtures for the diabetic

Some diabetics need to be careful, especially when taking cough mixtures containing syrup, as these may affect efficient diabetic (blood sugar) control. Many cough medicines today come in special forms suitable for the diabetic patient, e.g. Codeine Linctus Diabetic, Pavacol-D, Pholcomed Forte Diabetic and Pholtex.

3

REMEDIES THAT SUPPRESS THE APPETITE

The idea of a remedy that will take away our appetite for food and thus allow us to slim easily is an attractive one. The medical profession has generally turned its back on the subject of slimming in this fashion, but a few doctors have gathered together an impressive retinue of patients who are delighted to slim with the aid of drugs. The history of slimming with the benefit of medicines is, unfortunately, littered with unsuccessful cures, and there is no doubt that quackery, both from within and outside the medical profession, sometimes relieves the gullible of their cash rather than their weight.

The whole matter has been made rather worse by the unfortunate, disinterested attitude of a large number of medical practitioners towards attempts to produce slimming aids. This has been compounded by a downright unscientific and totally critical approach to those that do exist. The aphorism that 'everything that is *you* has come off a plate or from a glass' is only true (if it is true at all) in a biologically controlled environment that has nothing to do with everyday life. Many half truths are masquerading as fundamental concepts and nutritional facts. The idea of giving calorific values to certain foods is convenient for the purposes of comparison. But it only gives the vaguest indication of the food's propensity to make anyone gain weight.

Whether or not an individual is gaining or losing weight does, of course, bear a relationship to the amount of food absorbed by the body. If more food is absorbed than the body needs at any time, then excess intake is likely to be reflected in increased weight. If less food is absorbed than the body needs, then this deficiency is reflected in a falling weight. The important thing to remember is that the body's needs for energy are highly idiosyncratic. For example, the fact that one car will run for thirty miles on a gallon of petrol and another for only fifteen, tells us something about the energy needs of various vehicles. In this simple concept we acknowledge that not all machines are equally efficient. The human machine is equally variable and it would be very curious if this were not so. This gives us a real insight into those two opposites in the world of weight control—Mr Fatten Easily and Mrs Constant Weight.

While still in the world of motoring, there are cars that go faster and go further, or both, than other cars. They use more fuel than those that clock up smaller and more leisurely mileages, of course. People are the same.

For years nutritionists have scoffed at the idea of exercise having much effect on weight control, because the human machine is so efficient. In other words it can do a lot of work on a small ration of fuel (food). This fallacy arose from measurements of energy consumption carried out by people in physiological laboratories. In such situations it is possible to measure quite accurately the energy consumed in various activities, like walking, running and so on. Calculations can then be designed that appear to show that to lose a little weight you would have to walk for instance from London to Brighton. These so-called facts are, in reality, fiction. They omit to take account of the existence of a type of 'knock-on' effect in exercise. A shortish period of activity, of course, consumes a short 'blast' of energy. This is what gets measured in the laboratory. But it does something else too. It resets the body's internal chemistry to work at an increased rate, and this increased rate persists for quite a long time *after* the exercise is over; this does not get measured by those white-coated scientists who work out energy-expenditure tables.

Finally, the antislimming-pill philosophy gets considerable support from doctors generally because *some* slimming pills are addictive or at least habit-forming. Doctors also have fairly entrenched (but often unsupported) opinions about slimming pill efficiency. Actually research supports the efficiency of many such pills and proves that slimmers using them lose more weight, in controlled circum-stances, than those taking placebo (dummy) tablets.

There is one more important fact to be realised by all who wish to lose weight and who look at the possibilities of appetite suppression as an aid. For sustained improvement on this score a modification has to be made in the slimmer's eating pattern and exercise lifestyle if a *permanent* rearrangement of body weight is to be the goal. Appetite suppressants can help, and do help, but they are slimming *aids* and not medical treatments in their own right.

Compound slimming remedies

Two groups of compounds to help slimming are available: bulk-forming substances; and drugs that act on the appetite-controlling centres in the brain (central action remedies).

BULK-FORMING SUBSTANCES

These substances work on the principle of providing a sensation of satiety. There are foodstuffs high in bulk, like raw celery, salad vegetables, or bran (both in the form of wholemeal bread, *All-Bran*, or 'pure' bran). These, taken in doses of 2 tablespoonfuls daily mixed with food, or by themselves, can often eliminate the need for medicines. Usually such foodstuffs act as mild laxatives and, because they stimulate rapid passage of food through the bowel, may produce wind, gas pains and mild colic for a week or so until they are better tolerated. There are no special precautions to be observed while using these products.

▲ **Celevac**

3 tablets chewed or crushed with half a pint of water half an hour before meals, or when hungry.

▲ Cellucon
1–4 tablets taken as for Celevac.

▲ Nilstim
2 tablets taken as for Celevac.

▲ Prefil
Two (5 ml) spoonfuls taken as for Celevac.

CENTRAL-ACTING REMEDIES

AMPHETAMINE (DEXAMPHETAMINE)
Dexedrine, Durophet
- *Basic precautions:* Dependence and tolerance occur rapidly. Not suitable for use by patients with heart disease or high blood pressure, thyroid disease, glaucoma or together with MAOI drugs.
- *Proper dosage:* Dexedrine—5 mg thrice daily taken twenty minutes before meals and not after 6 pm. Durophet—manufactured in three capsule strengths. 1 capsule at breakfast (capsule is compounded with a resin complex to provide slow release).
- *Side effects:* Dryness of mouth, agitation, insomnia, palpitation, tremor.
- *Special advantages:* Only acceptable as a short-term introduction to a reducing regime. Weight loss occurs even on 'free-eating' regimen.

DIETHYLPROPION
Apisate (contains vitamins), Tenuate Dospan
- *Basic precautions:* Not suitable for patients with hypertension, heart disease, angina, peptic ulcer, diabetes, glaucoma, thyroid disease, or those on MAOI drugs, or within two weeks of taking these. Not to be used by the emotionally unstable, or those susceptible to dependence (although this is rare).
- *Proper dosage:* Apisate and Tenuate Dospan. Depends on eating habits—1 sustained-release tablet produces a ten-hour effect on appetite. A period of six to eight weeks' treatment is suggested, followed by four weeks free of treatment. If necessary, the patient may then resume dosage.
- *Special advantages:* Although this belongs to the amphetamine family, chemically this drug produces few dependence problems. However, excessive abuse has produced serious psychological problems. A useful and generally safe aid to weight control.

FENFLURAMINE
Ponderax, Pacaps (one of several preparations; sustained-release form)
- *Basic precautions:* Not to be taken in conjunction with or within three weeks of MAOI drugs. To be used with caution for persons suffering from depression. Sometimes impairment of concentration and difficulty in operating machinery occurs.
- *Proper dosage:* For mild obesity—20 mg twice daily in the first week, then 20 mg thrice daily. Moderate obesity—20 mg twice daily in the first week, then 40 mg twice daily. Severe obesity—20 mg twice daily in the first week, then 40 mg thrice daily. Pacaps—1–2 capsules once daily as prescribed, taken half an hour before food. Long-term medication possible.

- *Side effects:* Gastrointestinal upset, sedation, dizziness, dry mouth, sleep disturbance. Rarely palpitation, hair loss, anaemia. Treatment should be terminated gradually to obviate a risk of withdrawal depression.
- *Special advantages:* Excellent for those who find this remedy suitable in terms of side effects. Can be used by them on a long-term basis.

MAZINDOL
Teronac

- *Basic precautions:* Not suitable for patients with peptic ulcer, glaucoma, severe kidney, liver, heart or blood pressure disease. Caution in the agitated or thyroid cases. Certain cough medicines are prohibited (those containing sympathomimetic drugs). May upset insulin requirements of diabetics. Caution needed while driving or operating machinery.
- *Proper dosage:* 1 tablet after breakfast, continued for three months in conjunction with suitable diet prescribed by the doctor.
- *Side effects:* Constipation, dry mouth, insomnia. Rarely nervousness, headache, dizziness, 'shivers', rashes, delay in urination and onset of ejaculation.
- *Special advantages:* Has a selective amphetamine-type effect on the appetite centre in the brain, but is unrelated chemically to such drugs.

PHENTERMINE
Duromine, Ionamin

- *Basic precautions:* Not to be used for patients with severe blood pressure, thyroid disease, agitation, depressive illness or with MAOI drugs and some blood pressure-reducing drugs (consult your doctor if you are taking these). Caution advised if taking certain cough and cold remedies.
- *Proper dosage:* Both drugs available in two strengths. 15–30 mg before breakfast, or ten to fourteen hours before bedtime.
- *Side effects:* Dryness of mouth, insomnia, palpitation. Rarely long-term depression.
- *Special advantages:* Produces less excitement than most amphetamine-type derivatives.

OTC slimming 'specialities'

The following products are available OTC and, if taken according to manufacturer's instructions, are safe concoctions.

PRE-MEAL AIDS

▲ Slim Line
A chewing gum containing benzocaine, which reduces the sense of taste, so lessening the craving for food.

▲ Ayds
Chewy cubes of glucose and vitamins, containing 25 calories per cube. 1 chewed before a meal acts as an appetite-controller, taking the edge off the appetite.

REPLACEMENT MEALS

These substitute meals give 160–250 calories per meal. They all consist of food mixtures, plus vitamins.

Biscuit types
▲ **Limmits, Crunch and Slim**

Liquid types
May be mixed with water or milk (less slimming) to make a drink.
▲ **Slimgard, HPD, Slender, Slim Plan**

Combined
▲ **Slimgard 5-Day Diet**
Biscuits, drink and in-between chews.

▲ **Lessen**
Biscuits and drink.

Soups
▲ **Slender Slim Soups**

Chocolate or crunchie bars
▲ **Slender Bars**

ARTIFICIAL SWEETENERS

SACCHARIN
▲ **Natrena, Hermesetas, Sweetex, Saxin** (in tablet, liquid and powder forms).

SACCHARIN AND SUGAR COMBINATIONS
▲ **Sucron, Suga Twin**
These look like sugar and since they are a mixture of sugar and saccharin, produce sugar-like flavour with fewer calories than plain sugar.

4

REMEDIES FOR THE CONTROL OF INFECTION

Many of the advances in medicine over the last twenty-five years have been in the control of infection. The doctor's task in this field is not easy, because one can either 'rush into antibiotics' or delay their prescription; each attitude holds its hazards. Happily in Britain all the major drugs used to control infection are available only on prescription and so we should be spared the inappropriate use of these valuable compounds. Unfortunately there are always those who will dip into a family member's prescription or 'finish up' some neighbour's left-over drugs and thus run into problems.

There is some evidence that neither medical nor patient mismanagement is entirely responsible for the less than satisfactory state of affairs in the control of infection today. More and more germs are learning to live with antibiotics, and it is highly likely that the ingenuity of nature rather than the mistakes of man is responsible: antibiotic-resistant strains of all sorts of common germs are emerging and making themselves very much felt in the world today.

Another aspect of the use of antibiotics is the plethora of side effects. This, added to the fact that the control of one type of germ within the body often acts as a stimulus to other organisms, often produces unwanted symptoms.

Some of these hazards can be minimised by observing carefully the instructions on the use of these drugs. Precise timing of regime and length of treatment are particularly important on this score.

Because of the very many drugs prescribed and available in this section, a rather different format of presentation is followed from the rest of the book. The various drugs will be classified as below:

The penicillins
The cephalosporins
The tetracyclines
Other antibiotics
The sulphonamides and co-trimoxazole
The treatment of tuberculosis
The antifungal remedies
Drugs active against viruses

A 'basic precautions' section may not always be relevant and so may not be mentioned. Injectable penicillins and other injectable drugs, being more strictly under medical control, are omitted from this summary entirely.

The penicillins

General note: There are particular side effects associated with these drugs. These include the itchy, lumpy rash of urticaria (hives), fever, joint pains and the rapid swelling of the tissues (often of the face) known as angioneurotic oedema. The most worrying reaction to all penicillins is a generalised reaction, the so-called anaphylactic shock reaction, in which breathing and cardiac problems predominate. These may, unless promptly dealt with, lead to collapse and even death. Sensitivity reactions are a general problem because, once a patient develops sensitivity to one penicillin, this generally speaking spreads to all penicillins.

Penicillins currently used

AMOXYCILLIN
Amoxil
- *Proper dosage (various preparations):* 250 mg every eight hours, taken before food; to be doubled in cases of severe infection.
- *Special advantages:* Well absorbed by mouth, producing high blood or tissue concentrations. Has a broad spectrum of activity.

Augmentin (amoxycillin plus clavulanic acid)
- *Proper dosage:* 1–2 tablets thrice daily for up to fourteen days.
- *Special advantages:* Useful in penicillin-resistant infections of urinary tract.

AMPICILLIN
Amfipen, Penbritin, Pentrexyl, Vidopen and Ampicillin (F)
- *Proper dosage (various preparations):* 0.25–1 g taken at least thirty minutes before food, every six hours.
- *Special advantages:* Less well absorbed than amoxycillin. Broad spectrum of activity.

BENZATHINE PENICILLIN
Penidural
- *Proper dosage (various preparations):* 450 mg every six to eight hours.
- *Special advantages:* Really these are *disadvantages*—absorption from gut is slow (best used by injection).

BENZYLPENICILLIN
Crystapen G
- *Proper dosage:* 250 mg every six hours.
- *Special advantages:* As for benzathine penicillin.

CARFECILLIN
Uticillin
- *Proper dosage:* 0.5–1 g thrice daily.
- *Special advantages:* Useful in special types of urinary infection.

CICLACILLIN
Calthor
- *Proper dosage:* 250–500 mg every six hours.
- *Special advantages:* Fairly well absorbed. Useful for bronchitis, urinary tract and soft tissue infection.

CLOXACILLIN
Orbenin, Ampliclox (cloxacillin and ampicillin)
- *Proper dosage:* 500 mg every six hours.
- *Special advantages:* Not inactivated by common penicillin-resistant organisms.

FLUCLOXACILLIN
Floxapen
- *Proper dosage:* 250 mg every six hours, taken at least thirty minutes before food.
- *Special advantages:* As for Orbenin, but twice as well absorbed.

FLUCLOXACILLIN + AMPICILLIN
Magnapen
- *Proper dosage:* 1 capsule or 10 ml of syrup four times daily, half to one hour before meals.
- *Special advantages:* Used in severe infections when penicillin-resistant germs are suspected.

PENAMECILLIN
Havapen
- *Proper dosage:* 350 mg thrice daily.
- *Special advantages:* Especially useful for penicillin-resistant germs in adults.

PHENETHICILLIN
Broxil (several preparations)
- *Proper dosage:* 250 mg every six hours.
- *Special advantages:* As for phenoxymethylpenicillin.

PHENOXYMETHYLPENICILLIN (PENICILLIN V)
Apsin VK, Crystapen V, Distaquaine VK, Icipen, Stabillin VK, V-Cil-K and Phenoxymethylpenicillin (F)
- *Proper dosage:* 250–500 mg every six hours, taken at least thirty minutes before food.
- *Special advantages:* Is acid stable so not easily destroyed by enzymes in the stomach; absorption is unpredictable and so this drug is not relied upon to treat serious infections when taken by mouth.

PIVAMPICILLIN
Pondocillin
- *Proper dosage:* 500 mg every twelve hours, doubled in cases of severe infection.
- *Special advantages:* As for ampicillin. Broad spectrum of activity.

TALAMPICILLIN
Talpen
- *Proper dosage:* 250–500 mg every eight hours.
- *Special advantages:* As for ampicillin, but better absorbed.

The cephalosporins

These antibiotics were developed to provide substitutes for penicillin when the latter became ineffective. They have been successful in this sphere to some extent. Hypersensitivity tends to limit the use of penicillins in certain people and the cephalosporins were seen as a way out of this dilemma. Unfortunately about 10 per cent of penicillin-sensitive patients are also sensitive to cephalosporins. The latter also have certain intrinsic health hazards linked to their use. The following review omits preparations that can only be used in injection form.

Penicillin substitutes commonly used

CEFACLOR
Distaclor
● *Basic precautions:* Caution advised if patient is penicillin-sensitive.
● *Proper dosage:* 250 mg every eight hours; increase if necessary, to maximum dosage of 2 g per day.
● *Side effects:* Allergic reactions, hypersensitivity (chest, heart or general symptoms), nausea, vomiting; diarrhoea is common.
● *Special advantages:* A broad-spectrum penicillin-like antibiotic.

CEPHALEXIN
Ceporex, Keflex and Cephalexin (F)
● *Basic precautions:* As for cefaclor; special care needed for patients with kidney problems. May produce false results in some urine tests.
● *Proper dosage:* 250–500 mg every six hours.
● *Side effects:* As for cefaclor.
● *Special advantages:* As for cefaclor.

CEPHRADINE
Velosef
Details: As for cephalexin.

The tetracyclines

These are broad-spectrum antibiotics that have certain advantages over the penicillins and cephalosporins because sensitivity reactions are rare. Unfortunately their very wide use has diminished their usefulness; as many of the bacteria that tetracycline was able to control have now developed resistance to its action. The tetracyclines do have certain inherent disadvantages; they are deposited in growing bone and teeth, causing staining and other dental problems in children. This prohibits their use for two large groups of people: children under the age of twelve and pregnant women. Absorption of the tetracyclines is diminished by milk and antacid mixtures and also some other medicines, especially those containing calcium, iron and magnesium. One constant hazard with tetracyclines is the encouragement of the secondary growth of various organisms present in the body —especially fungus and yeast organisms. The use of the tetracyclines may therefore precipitate attacks of thrush in various forms.

Apart from dosages there is little to choose between tetracyclines as far as their use is concerned, and so no individual schedules will be given.

Drugs commonly used

Active principal	Proprietary preparation	Formulary preparation	Dosage
Chlortetracycline	Aureomycin		250–500 mg six-hourly
Clomocycline	Megaclor		170–340 mg six-hourly
Demeclocycline	Ledermycin		150 mg six-hourly
Doxycycline	Vibramycin*		200 mg on first day followed by 100 mg daily
Lymecycline	Tetralysal		408 mg every twelve hours
Methacycline	Rondomycin		150 mg every six hours
Minocycline	Minocin†		200 mg initially, then 100 mg twice daily
Oxytetracycline	Berkmycen Chemocycline Galenomycin Imperacin Oxymycin Terramycin Unimycin	Oxytetracycline	250–500 mg six-hourly
Tetracycline	Achromycin Deteclo Economycin Sustamycin Tetrabid Tetrachel Tetrex	Tetracycline	250–500 mg six-hourly

General note: These preparations are available in various forms—tablets, capsules and syrups. In many cases the main difference lies in the price and the flavour of liquid preparations. Exceptions to this appraisal are claimed by various manufacturers. The following are well-acknowledged exceptions: *Vibramycin—a well-tolerated, once-a-day preparation, which does not produce kidney problems; †Minocin—has a somewhat broader spectrum of activity than most tetracyclines. In practice some minor variations of dosages in certain preparations may be recommended.

- *Basic precautions:* Not suitable for patients with kidney failure, pregnant women especially, and children under twelve. Can cause photosensitivity (skin sunlight reaction).
- *Side effects:* Nausea, vomiting, diarrhoea, superinfection with other organisms.
- *Special advantages:* Very effective broad range of antibacterial activity. The tetracyclines are used locally in many ointments and are taken by mouth for many skin diseases. (*See* Chapter 6, page 83.)

Combination products

Combination products tend to have hazards as well as advantages attached to their use, but some drugs are fairly frequently used and deserve mention. Their components determine side effects, dosage and advantages. All products are available on prescription only.

OXYTETRACYCLINE AND BROMHEXINE
Bisolvomycin
A mucolytic product which aids the liquification of mucus. Special care for patients with peptic ulcer. Dosage: 1 capsule four times daily.

TETRACYCLINE AND NYSTATIN
Mysteclin
An antifungal antibiotic and broad-spectrum antibiotic. Can be used by patients who may not otherwise be prescribed such drugs. Dosage: 250 mg six-hourly.

OXYTETRACYCLINE, EPHEDRINE AND IPECACUANHA
Terra-Bron
A breathing-tube antispasmodic and expectorant. Dosage: 5 ml taken six-hourly. Not suitable for patients with heart failure, hypertension, thyroid or prostatic disease.

Other antibiotics

Research has been active in producing new and very specialised preparations. For instance, streptomycin is almost entirely reserved for the treatment of tuberculosis. Some antibiotics are used entirely by injection or in intravenous therapy and are not within the scope of this book. Some antibiotics are applied locally to the skin, either alone or with other medicaments; these may be gentamycin, neomycin and framycetin and though they are active against many invading organisms they can cause problems of sensitivity. Antibiotics can also be toxic in their own right and are thus kept for the management of serious conditions that might not otherwise be controlled; such drugs as clindamycin sodium fusidate (Fucidin) and chloramphenicol. Some of these, however, may be used quite safely on the skin (*see* Chapter 6).

One of the most helpful of this group of remedies in this section is erythromycin.

ERYTHROMYCIN
Erycen, Erythrocin, Erythromid, Erythroped, Ilosone, Ilotycin, Retcin
- *Basic precautions:* Not suitable for patients who have previously had jaundice or who are known to have liver disease.
- *Proper dosage (various preparations):* 250–500 mg every six hours.
- *Side effects:* Mild nausea and vomiting, and sometimes acute diarrhoea. Very rarely a form of hepatitis (with or without jaundice) occurs; this is signalled by malaise, nausea, vomiting, colic and fever. This is always an indication to stop treatment. Generally such problems only occur after one to two weeks' therapy. Symptoms stop on cessation of treatment but will reappear if drug is taken again.
- *Special advantages:* A useful alternative to penicillin in hypersensitive patients. May be a useful prophylactic in whooping cough.

The sulphonamides and co-trimoxazole

An historical perspective will enhance our understanding of the way the drugs of this particular group work. During the Second World War the early sulphonamides, especially sulphapyridine (such as M & B 693) gave the first glimpse of the antibiotic era that was to follow. While the sulphonamides ('sulfa drugs') were not antibiotics, they did stop certain bacteria from multiplying within the body. They are therefore called bacteriostatics. A new development in this field has been to combine a sulphonamide with another compound (trimethoprim) in the form of co-trimoxazole. This allows sulphonamides to become bacteriocidal rather than bacteriostatic. So successful has this combination been that co-trimoxazole has become the prime example of modern sulphonamide therapy, and apart from a handful of 'specialised' sulphonamides, has largely replaced them in general use.

Drugs commonly used

Active principal	Proprietary preparation	Type	Formulary preparation
Calcium Sulphaloxate	Enteromide	PA	
Co-trimoxazole	Bactrim Septrin	FAA	Co-trimoxazole tablets and mixtures
Phthalysulphathiazole	Thalazole	PA	
Sulfametopyrazine	Kelfizine W	U/C	
Sulphadiazine	Streptotriad Sulphatriad	G G	
Sulphadimethoxine	Madribon	U/C	
Sulphadimidine	Sulphamezathine	U	
Sulphafurazole	Gantrisin	U	
Sulphaguanidine		PA	Sulphaguanidine tablets
Sulphamethizole	Urolucosil	U	Sulphamethizole tablets
Sulphamethoxypyridazine	Lederkyn	U	
Sulphapyridine	M & B 693	S	
Sulphathiazole	Thiazamide	G	
Sulphaurea	Uromide	U	

Key: FAA = folic acid antagonist sulphonamides; PA = poorly absorbed sulphonamides; U/C = urinary and chest infection; U = urinary tract infection; G = general-use sulphonamides; S = specialised-use sulphonamides.

Because the type of action provided by the sulphonamide—or the part of the body affected—is the single most important factor, the drugs listed above are now grouped into their key types for further analysis.

FOLIC ACID ANTAGONIST SULPHONAMIDES (FAA)

CO-TRIMOXAZOLE

Bactrim, Septrin

- *Basic precautions:* Not suitable for patients with liver damage, jaundice, severe kidney damage, or sensitivity to any sulphonamide or trimethoprim. Care needed with patients on oral diabetic drugs, or certain anticoagulants and for the elderly. Regular blood tests mandatory for long-term therapy.
- *Proper dosage:* There are several forms of preparation. For co-trimoxazole a schedule of at least five days' treatment (or two days after symptoms are relieved) is mandatory. For some chronic conditions prolonged treatment is necessary. The usual dosage is 2 tablets twice daily, reduced to 1 tablet daily if course of treatment exceeds fourteen days. For severe infections longer doses may be prescribed.
- *Side effects:* Nausea, vomiting, sore mouth, rashes. Treatments should be stopped if rash occurs. Blood disease is a rare side effect.
- *Special advantages:* Especially effective in urinary tract infections, prostatitis and certain chronic chest infections.

POORLY-ABSORBED SULPHONAMIDES (PA)

Active principal	Proprietary preparation	Dosage
Calcium sulphaloxate	Enteromide	2 tablets thrice daily
Phthalysulphathiazole	Thalazole	2–12 g daily in divided doses
Sulphaguanidine		3 g every eight hours for three days, then 3 g every twelve hours for four days

- *Basic precautions:* Not suitable for patients with sulphonamide sensitivity. Blood tests mandatory in long-term use.
- *Side effects:* As for co-trimoxazole, but milder.
- *Special advantages:* Sometimes helpful in bowel infections. Slight absorption from gut occurs, so few sensitivity problems.

URINARY TRACT AND CHEST INFECTION SULPHONAMIDES (U/C)

Active principal	Proprietary preparation	Dosage
Sulphadimethoxine	Madribon	1–2 g initially, then 500 mg daily
Sulfametopyrazine	Kelfizine W	2 g once weekly

- *Basic precautions:* As for co-trimoxazole. Adequate fluid intake needed for a week after treatment. Potassium citrate mixture must be taken concurrently with Kelfizine W.
- *Side effects:* As for co-trimoxazole; passing blood in urine is a rare side effect.
- *Special advantages:* Long-acting, low-dosage sulphonamides.

URINARY TRACT SULPHONAMIDES (U)

Active principal	Proprietary preparation	Dosage
Sulphadimidine	**Sulphamezathine**	2 g initially, then 0.5 g six-hourly
Sulphafurazole	**Gantrisin**	2 g initially, then 1 g six-hourly
Sulphamethizole	**Urolucosil**	200 mg five times daily
Sulphamethoxypyridazine	**Lederkyn**	1–2 g initially, then 500 mg daily
Sulphaurea	**Uromide**	2 dragees thrice daily

- *Basic precautions:* As for co-trimoxazole.
- *Side effects:* As for co-trimoxazole.
- *Special advantages:* Specially suitable for urinary tract problems.

GENERAL-USE SULPHONAMIDES (G)

Active principal	Proprietary preparations	Dosage
Sulphadiazine	**Streptotriad*** **Sulphatriad**†	2 tablets thrice daily 4 tablets initially, then 2 six-hourly (suspension: 5 ml = 1 tablet)
Sulphathiazole	**Thiazamide**	2 g initially, then 1 g six-hourly

* Contains other sulphonamides and streptomycin.
† Contains other sulphonamides.

- *Basic precautions:* As for co-trimoxazole.
- *Side effects:* As for co-trimoxazole.
- *Special advantages:* Streptotriad is used as a poorly-absorbed bowel sterilisation sulphonamide. The other compounds are little used today.

SPECIALISED-USE SULPHONAMIDES (S)

SULPHAPYRIDINE

Sulphapyridine
The original M & B 693, this drug is used for a rare skin disease (dermatitis herpetiformis).

- *Proper dosage:* 3–4 g daily until response is obtained; then 0.5–1 g daily.
- *Other details:* As for co-trimoxazole.

Treating tuberculosis

Until the coming of age of antibiotics, tuberculosis was attended by a threat to life or chronic disability. The development of antituberculosis drugs made a dramatic difference to this distressing situation. Even so, treatment has to be careful and thorough and many patients worry about the complexity and the apparently strenuous discipline of treatment. Quite often a complex drug programme is deemed mandatory. Unless patients understand why this is so, treatment schedules are not adhered to; this can create disappointing and possibly dangerous results.

Tuberculosis has taught physicians a great deal about antibiotics in general and one thing in particular. If antibiotics are used in a long-term context, the bacteria that they are supposed to be destroying eventually learn to live in their presence. In certain diseases and conditions in which antibiotics are used doctors first assess if the germ they are trying to eradicate is likely to respond to the antibiotic they have in mind. In other words it is ascertained whether the organism is sensitive to particular antibiotics. In many cases a simple and quick test can decide the issue. In tuberculosis, however, tests of sensitivity take several months to show positive results; therefore, instead of delaying treatment to await results of sensitivity tests, a 'block-buster' approach to treatment is not only justifiable, but may be mandatory. Two block-buster techniques are generally used.

Because tuberculosis treatment is so specialised, general principles of treatment only are discussed.

PHASE I

Treatment usually involves the daily use of isoniazid (**Rimifon**) and rifampicin (**Rifadin, Rimactane**) supplemented by ethambutol (**Myambutol**) or streptomycin. There are various combination remedies available that avoid some multiple-tablet-swallowing regimes. This treatment is continued until drug sensitivity results are known, which takes at least eight weeks.

PHASE II

Unless contraindications become evident, isoniazid is continued along with a second drug. This may be rifampicin, ethambutol, or other remedy such as capreomycin (**Capastat**), cycloserine, pyrazinamide (**Zinamide**). This phase of treatment lasts about nine months.

The whole area of the management of side effects and contraindications is not explored in this book. Due to the potentially serious nature of the disease the patient may have to accept a degree of drug reaction in order to overcome a life-threatening illness. Treatment schedules, in any case, have to be carefully monitored in a hospital or clinic.

Fungal infection treatment

Fungus infections can occur in various situations in the body—the skin, the reproductive tract, the bowel being common sites. A variety of antifungal drugs have evolved that are especially suited to certain types of infection and references to them will occur in Chapter 7 (*Disorders of sexual function*) and Chapter 6 (*Remedies used for the skin*).

In some cases the presence of a fungal infection implies an impaired immunity to the infecting agent. This may be secondary to disease or brought about by therapy. Some fungal infections result from antibiotic treatment, probably due to ecological factors operating locally. The following review does not include intravenous therapy.

Common fungal drugs and usages

Active principal	Usage	Proprietary preparation	Formulary preparation
Amphotericin	M/V/S	Fungilin suspension lozenges cream pessaries	
Clotrimazole	V S	Canesten duopack ▲ Canesten cream	
Econazole	V/S V S	Ecostatin Gyno-Pevaryl Pevaryl	
Griseofulvin	M M	Fulcin Grisovin	Griseofulvin
Ketoconazole	M	Nizoral	
Miconazole	M/S V V	▲ Daktarin oral gel Daktarin tablets Gyno-Daktarin pessaries combipack tampons ▲ Monistat cream and pessaries	Miconazole vaginal cream and pessaries
Natamycin	M/V/S	Pimafucin suspension cream vaginal tablets	
Nystatin	M/V/S	Nystan suspension tablets vaginal cream pessaries triple pack Nystavescent	

Key: M = mouth; V = vagina; S = skin.

AMPHOTERICIN

Fungilin

- *Basic precautions:* None.
- *Proper usage:* Cream and ointment—apply 2–4 times daily. Lozenges—1 dissolved in mouth four to eight times daily. Suspension—1 ml placed in mouth and kept in contact with tissues as long as possible. Tablets—1–2 tablets four times daily. Pessaries—1–2 pessaries inserted into vagina for fourteen consecutive nights.
- *Side effects:* None, except for tablets if given in high doses—causes mild gastro-intestinal upset.
- *Special advantages:* Active against wide range of yeasts and yeast-like fungi.

CLOTRIMAZOLE

Canesten duopack
▲ Canesten cream

- *Basic precautions:* None.
- *Proper usage:* Cream—apply thinly and rub in gently thrice daily for one month (or for two weeks after skin appears normal). Atomiser—use as for cream. Powder—sprinkle on after cream or atomiser usage. Vaginal tablets—two 100 mg

or one 200 mg inserted at night for three consecutive nights or one 500 mg as a single treatment. Vaginal cream—1 filled applicator twice daily for three consecutive days, or once daily for six consecutive nights. Duopack—tablets used as above and the cream applied at night and morning to sexual skin of both partners.

- *Side effects:* Slight local burning or irritation.
- *Special advantages:* A broad-spectrum antifungal—also active against trichomonas infection (TV).

ECONAZOLE
Ecostatin, Gyno-Pevaryl, Pevaryl
- *Basic precautions:* None, except keep away from eyes, and do not spray on mucous membrane.
- *Proper usage:* Application of various preparations twice daily. Pessaries—to be used nightly for three nights. Ecostatin twin pack—male partner should also use cream.
- *Side effects:* Rare itching and discomfort.
- *Special advantages:* Quick-acting, broad-spectrum antifungal; also effective against yeasts, and athlete's foot/tinea infections.

GRISEOFULVIN
Fulcin, Grisovin and Griseofulvin (F)
- *Basic precautions:* Not suitable for patients with severe liver disease or the rare condition, porphyria. May decrease effect of anticoagulants. Absorption inhibited by phenobarbitone. In rare cases can cause drowsiness; may potentiate alcohol.
- *Proper dosage:* 500–1000 mg per day. Treatment for hair or skin should be for at least four weeks; for nails six weeks' to two months' treatment may be necessary. Treatment continued for two weeks after apparent return to normalcy.
- *Side effects:* Headache, gastric discomfort, rashes.
- *Special advantages:* Penetrates to deep tissues and prevents newly-formed tissues being attacked by fungi.

KETOCONAZOLE
Nizoral
- *Basic precautions:* Not to be used with drugs that reduce stomach acid secretion. Not to be used during pregnancy.
- *Proper dosage:* 200 mg twice daily with meals for five days. Prophylaxis—1 daily.
- *Side effects:* Occasional nausea, rash, headache.

MICONAZOLE
▲ Daktarin, Monistat
Gyno-Daktarin and Miconazole (F)
- *Basic precautions:* None.
- *Proper dosage:* Daktarin tablets—1 tablet four times daily taken after meals. Should be continued for two days after symptoms have cleared. Used to eradicate fungus from bowel. Daktarin oral gel—1–2 teaspoonfuls kept in mouth for as long as possible, four times daily. Length of treatment as for tablets. Daktarin twin pack (cream and powder)—cream applied twice daily (once daily to nails and covered with occlusive dressing). Powder applied to clothes/shoes in contact with affected skin. Treatment to continue for ten days after apparent cure. Gyno-Daktarin

intravaginal cream and tampons, pessaries, combipack (cream and pessaries)—used nightly for seven nights. Cream and 2 pessaries at night, tampons night and morning. Monistat cream and pessaries, used nightly for fourteen nights. Miconazole cream and pessaries as directed.

● *Side effects:* Few, occasional irritation.
● *Special advantages:* Quick-acting, no side effects and wide range of products.

NATAMYCIN
Pimafucin
● *Basic precautions:* None.
● *Proper usage:* Suspension—10 drops taken by mouth after meals. Cream—apply thrice daily. Vaginal tablets—use nightly for twenty-one days.
● *Side effects:* Rarely irritation.

NYSTATIN
Nystan, Nystavescent
● *Basic precautions:* None.
● *Proper usage:* Nystan oral suspension—1 ml only held in mouth for as long as possible four times daily. Tablets—1 tablet four times daily. Cream, ointment, gel, dusting powder—apply 2–4 times daily. Vaginal pessaries (Nystan and Nysta-vescent)—1–2 inserted for fourteen nights. Vaginal cream—1–2 applications in vagina for fourteen nights. (Treat male concurrently with gel in coital situation.)
● *Side effects:* Negligible; tablets may cause mild gastrointestinal upsets.
● *Special advantages:* Wide range of products.

The development of drugs active against viruses

Until comparatively recently viral infections were the Cinderella of therapy. This was because suitable medicines that killed viruses, and left the rest of the body intact, defied development. The success stories of medicine versus virus come from the world of preventative medicine—vaccines for polio, smallpox, rubella and to some extent influenza are examples of this. In certain other diseases vaccines are therapeutic, as is the case in rabies. Temporary immunity against the virus's action on the body can be 'bought' by means of an injection of a non-specific substance called gamma-globulin which is widely used in prophylaxis for rubella and infective hepatitis.

Gradually, however, potent and specific antivirus 'antibiotics' have been developed. Three such sbstances in use today, are discussed in this book. Others are being developed or are given exclusively by injection.

Three antiviral drugs

Active principal	Proprietary preparation	Sphere of use
Acyclovir	Zovirax	Herpes infections
Amantadine	Symmetrel	Prophylaxis influenza Treatment of shingles
Idoxuridine	Herpid	Herpes zoster (shingles)

ACYCLOVIR
Zovirax
At the time of writing this compound is in the process of being introduced into the pharmacopoeia. It seems to be a very effective remedy against the herpes virus in all its forms. It can be taken by mouth or applied to herpes lesions (cold sores, eye herpes, genital herpes) locally, in the form of ointment. To be effective the drug has to be taken as early as possible in the development of symptoms. In herpes on the face or sexual skin, in most cases there are well marked *prodromal* symptoms. In other words the skin that is to develop the herpes rash becomes itchy, sore or feels prickly. If the ointment is rubbed in at this stage thrice daily, for five to seven days, most outbreaks of herpes can be prevented. More important perhaps, the patient is not infectious to others. There appear to be no side effects or special precautions to be observed.

AMANTADINE
Symmetrel
(Also used in the treatment of Parkinson's disease, *see* page 174.)
- *Basic precautions:* Not suitable for patients who are subject to convulsions or who have a history of gastric ulceration. Special care needed for the confused patient or those subject to hallucinations. Caution advised in use for patients with kidney disease.
- *Proper dosage:* For herpes zoster (shingles)—1 capsule twice daily for fourteen days. If pain persists treatment is extended for a further fourteen days. For influenza (A$_2$ strain)—for prophylaxis 1 capsule twice daily for as long as protection is required (usually seven to ten days); for treatment 1 capsule twice daily for five to seven days.
- *Side effects:* Possible side effects include swelling of fingers, toes, face and rashes, More rarely nervousness, insomnia, dizziness, convulsions or hallucinations.
- *Special advantages:* Useful addition to therapy for diseases for which no other specific treatment is available.

IDOXURIDINE
Herpid
- *Basic precautions:* None, though strict attention to duration of treatment is necessary.
- *Proper usage:* Solution to be painted on skin lesions and around their base four times daily, for four days.
- *Side effects:* Local stinging and sometimes a distinctive taste in mouth. Contact may damage synthetic materials.
- *Special advantages:* A good remedy if used as early as possible in painful and unpleasant conditions.

5

TREATING DISEASES OF THYROID FUNCTION

Self-medication has no real role to play in this particular illness, since all medication is prescription only. But it is necessary to understand the general principles that underlie treatment of thyroid malfunction. This is because once treatment is initiated (usually at a hospital level), it has to be maintained on a long-term basis if a reasonable state of health is to be expected.

The thyroid gland, located in the neck, is primarily involved in metabolism (the use of energy in the body), which it affects by producing iodine-containing hormones. This hormone production can go awry in two ways. There may be a deficiency in hormone production or the hormones may be produced to excess. The former problem occurs in two main forms.

Thyroid hormone deficiency disease

I Caused by *blocked* hormone production
The interference in hormone production is of two kinds. In one instance it is a nutritional defect: the body does not have enough of the element iodine to build the essential hormone. When this occurs the thyroid gland tends to become enlarged in its attempt to produce more hormone. In this condition, a *simple* goitre develops in the neck (the relevance of the word 'simple' will be obvious in a few moments). There are several reasons why goitres develop.

Dietary goitres occurred in the past, in areas located away from the coast, where the water or diet lacks iodine. The classic example was in Derbyshire where 'Derbyshire neck' was common. Addition of iodine to table salt has, generally speaking, prevented this disease, but there are certain hard-water areas where a high level of calcium effectively 'blocks' iodine absorption. It would seem that certain folk have an inherent difficulty in producing enough thyroid hormone and so become goitreous.

There is also what might be looked upon as self-induced goitre. Iodine mixtures —once popular for coughs—paramino-salicylic acid (used in the treatment of tuberculosis) and the sulphonamide drugs can interfere with thyroid hormone production and produce goitre, if they are used over a long period. It has even been reported that certain foodstuffs—if taken in large quantities by vegetarians—

(particularly cabbage, Brussel sprouts and turnips) can block thyroid hormone production. Modern treatment of goitre is usually based on prescribing synthetic thyroid hormone which also reduces the gland's overgrowth. This is known as thyroid replacement therapy.

II Caused by *low* hormone production
In this case the thyroid gland just does not work properly because of a variety of reasons. A variety of illnesses can be caused by low hormone production, including *cretinism* (the result of a congenital non-functioning gland) and various forms of *myxoedema* in which the gland malfunctions. Long-term replacement regimes based on synthetic thyroid hormone is effective treatment.

Overaction of the thyroid gland

The thyroid gland, in some conditions, seems to gear itself for overactivity. In order to do this it often becomes enlarged; thus the so-called *toxic goitre* occurs in the neck. This disease is called thyrotoxicosis. We do not know exactly how it is caused but treatment involves drugs which inhibit hormone production. These can be either special antithyroid drugs or radioactive drugs; surgeons can also remove a portion of the overactive gland. The management of thyrotoxicosis is always a delicate matter, needing fine judgment for the best results. Even so, because the symptoms of thyrotoxicosis are often so alarming, and on occasion possibly dangerous, attempts to control the hormone production may well damage the gland permanently and to such an extent that its vital function is impaired after treatment. When this happens a lifetime of synthetic hormone-taking becomes the lot of the patient cured of a toxic thyroid.

THYROID REPLACEMENT THERAPY

Years ago remedies made from the dried gland of various animals were the only means of administering replacement therapy. Unfortunately, like most biological products of this nature, the preparations were unstable and their action unpredictable. Now, new standardised preparations have replaced them. These are only available on prescription.

Preparations commonly used

THYROXINE SODIUM
Eltroxin and Thyroxine tablets (F)
- *Basic precautions:* Especial care needed for use of either drug by cardiac patients; an ECG is mandatory before treatment commences.
- *Proper dosage:* Patients over fifty usually start on 25–50 micrograms daily, taken before breakfast, increasing after one month to 50–75 micrograms (daily), and thereafter increasing by 25 micrograms every four weeks. Younger patients start at 50–100 micrograms daily, taken before breakfast, adjusted by 50 micrograms at three- to four-weekly intervals until required effect maintained. Physician will adjust dosage to match clinical improvement and control side effects. Special routines are necessary for infants and children.
- *Side effects:* Chest pain, palpitation, cramp, diarrhoea, restlessness, excitability, headache, face flushing, sweating, excessive weight loss and muscular weakness.

● *Special advantages:* The usual first choice for maintenance therapy.

Tertroxin
● *Basic precautions:* As for thyroxine sodium.
● *Proper dosage:* The drug may be prescribed for several problems. Thyroid deficiency—10–20 micrograms, increasing to 20–30 micrograms daily after one week, and thereafter adjusted by 10 micrograms every seven days. Elderly patients need half the dosage. Thyrotoxicosis (for replacement therapy)—80 micrograms per day.
● *Side effects:* As for thyroxine sodium.
● *Special advantages:* This may be looked upon as a rapid action and rapidly excreted form of thyroxine sodium. It is especially valuable in the treatment of severe thyroid deficiency and as a replacement remedy after, or together with, thyroid activity lowering treatments (ie for thyrotoxicosis).

ANTITHYROID DRUGS

CARBIMAZOLE
Neo-Mercazole
● *Basic precautions:* A close doctor–patient relationship is mandatory in order to anticipate possibly serious side effects.
● *Proper dosage:* 10–15 mg eight-hourly until patient is judged by doctor to be non-toxic. Dose then reduced to maintenance level of 5–15 mg per day. If rashes occur, propylthiouracil should be substituted (100–150 mg eight-hourly). During the treatment phase it is important to space out dosage evenly over the twenty-four-hour period. Once maintenance doses are reached a once-daily regime is allowed.
● *Side effects:* Side effects have to be differentiated from overdosage, in which signs of thyroid deficiency develop (tiredness, lethargy, gruffness of voice, increase in weight). Side effects include rashes, nausea, headache, aching joints, gastric upsets, and rarely hair loss. These usually occur during first eight weeks of treatment and are self-limiting. Should sore throat or fever develop, this may indicate damage to blood-forming mechanisms and treatment must be stopped. Usually one to two years' treatment is necessary.
● *Special advantages:* A well-tried and safe drug in most cases which can obviate the necessity of operation or radioactive treatment.

IODINE
Aqueous iodine solution
● *Basic precautions:* Not advisable if there is previous known iodine sensitivity. Not to be given to patients treated with potassium perchlorate.
● *Proper dosage:* 0.5 ml thrice daily, for two weeks prior to operation.
● *Side effects:* Symptoms of a cold, headache, pain in face and neck, rashes, chest and larynx irritation.

POTASSIUM PERCHLORATE
Peroidin
● *Basic precautions:* Not suitable for treatment of enlarged thyroid.

- *Proper dosage:* 200–250 mg every six to eight hours. Maximum dosage 1 g per day; reduce to 100–125 mg every six to eight hours after two to four weeks.
- *Side effects:* Gastrointestinal upset, rashes. Fever, anaemia, or body swelling are danger signals.
- *Special advantages:* May be useful if other antithyroid drugs cannot be used, but caution must be maintained in case blood-forming tissues are damaged.

PROPYLTHIOURACIL

Propylthiouracil tablets (F)

- *Basic precautions:* As for carbimazole.
- *Proper dosage:* 100–150 mg eight-hourly.
- *Side effects:* As for carbimazole.
- *Special advantages:* May be used when carbimazole side effects are unacceptable. Rarely damages blood-forming tissues.

Chapter

6

REMEDIES USED FOR
THE SKIN

The skin is, in fact, the largest organ of the body. Because it is so familiar to us this organ's functions are generally overlooked—we think of it essentially as a body covering and we say, of course, that beauty is skin deep. However, to understand how remedies and treatments affect the skin, it is worthwhile remembering a few simple facts about its function.

The skin and the nervous system arise from the self-same cells in the developing baby. This link is maintained throughout life and so certain upsets or derangements of the nervous system, such as anxiety and stress, may produce or aggravate changes in the skin. Eczema and dermatitis are cases in point. The nature of this two-way link is sometimes important to the understanding of side effects resulting from the use of skin remedies.

The skin also acts as a major body temperature control organ, and so problems of temperature regulation can produce skin trouble, eg prickly heat and intertrigo (a skin-rubbing problem). In addition, skin must be lubricated, otherwise it would graze very easily. The grease produced by the skin glands (sebaceous glands) performs this function. These glands are affected in turn by sex hormone changes, and this connection leads to sex hormone-related skin problems (eg acne).

The commonly acknowledged function of our skin—to cover us—leads in turn to many of the common skin problems that flesh is heir to: infection, sensitivity, damage from chemicals, or from light. The fact that the skin is the major contact point between *us* and a possibly hostile environment has led to defence (immune) systems being located in the skin. Disturbances and strange responses from our skin's defence systems are manifested quite often as skin allergy, rashes and so on.

Finally, the skin is, like any other tissue in the body, subject to certain unique diseases. These include psoriasis, warts and corns. It also bears hairs which may cause special problems (eg boils).

Happily, the skin is very amenable to local treatment. This is because the target tissue involved in a skin problem can be placed in intimate contact with medication. But there is a tendency, when using local treatments, to use too little or too much medication or to forget doses—or sometimes stop treatment too soon because the skin 'looks better'. Really effective skin treatment means being as careful about prescribed dosages as with other forms of therapy.

One important aspect of all skin medication is concerned with the formulation of the ointment, cream or lotion. The 'vehicle'—the substance that 'carries' the drug to be used—is often as important as the drug itself. When deciding on the vehicle to be used, manufacturers are careful to consider things like acceptability to the user, smell and cosmetic effect, as well as safety and stability. Doctors and skin specialists are stressing today that the 'vehicle' in skin treatments is often as important as the medication it contains. This is one reason why there are so many compounded preparations available for the treatment of skin problems—and the fact that one may suit the patient very much better than another in many cases. Quite often the most effective treatment can only be ultimately decided on a trial and error basis.

General note: In this chapter basic precautions and side effects are only noted where specifically applicable.

Skin cleaning, shampoos and antiseptics

(*See also* eczema and psoriasis treatments, page 95)

In some scaling disorders of the skin (certain forms of eczema, dermatitis, dandruff), cleansing preparations that are ideally non-irritant are prescribed—sometimes in the form of shampoos. The skin may also have to be cleaned after injury. In fact, efficient skin cleansing of cuts and grazes often means that the use of antiseptics is not necessary. In some cases a skin antiseptic is useful—for disinfecting cuts or blisters, cleaning around boils and other infected areas. The best skin antiseptics should not damage healing tissues, cause sensitivity reactions or destroy normal skin resistance. Such high treatment ideals, however, are rarely met in practice.

SKIN CLEANERS AND SHAMPOOS

ARACHIS OIL/LIQUID PARAFFIN

▲ **Oilatum emollient** (liquid paraffin in emulsion form)

▲ **Oilatum cream** (arachis oil in cream form)

▲ **Emulsifying ointment** (a mixture of liquid and soft paraffin with an emulsifying wax)

- *Basic precautions:* Always use with water: either apply to wet skin or add to bath or washing water. Beware of the possibility of slipping in the bath.
- *Proper usage:* Arachis oil/liquid paraffin and oilatum cream—add 1–3 capfuls to eight-inch bathwater or $\frac{1}{2}$–2 capfuls to baby's bath. Soak up to twenty minutes.
- *Special advantages:* Clears skin in conditions where ordinary soaps produce irritation. Prevents undue loss of skin oil and calms tense patients by soothing their skin.

CETRIMIDE

▲ **Savlon, Cetavlon, Propa PH**

(Cetrimide is the powder base of Cetavlon preparations. There are multiple products. Dissolved in water it is Cetavlon solution.)

- *Basic precautions:* Apply only locally to skin. Keep away from eyes; do not use in vaginal douche or enema; do not use to disinfect or clean syringes.

● *Proper usage:* Savlon and Cetavlon—a 1 per cent solution should be used for cleaning of skin crusts and scabs or to prevent infection. A 0.05 per cent solution should be used for final dip of nappies to prevent nappy rash. Cetavlon PC—used as a shampoo, should be diluted with ten parts of water. Shampoo carefully avoiding eyes. Cetavlon cream—designed to be applied to infected cuts or to burns.

● *Side effects:* Sensitivity reactions are rare.

COAL TAR

General note: Coal tar is the active principal and is combined with other substances.

▲ Alphosyl

(Multiple products. Contains coal tar and allantoin.)

● *Basic precautions:* For external use only.

● *Proper usage:* Massage gently into skin two to four times daily.

● *Side effects:* Sensitivity reactions are rare.

● *Special advantages:* The lotion is designed especially for psoriasis of skin and scalp. The cream is meant for lubricating skin-friction areas. Application PC shampoo used for psoriasis and dandruff.

▲ Polytar

(A mixture of various tars, arachis oil and liquid paraffin. Multiple products.)

● *Basic precautions:* Beware of slipping in the bath.

● *Proper usage:* 2–4 capfuls added to eight-inch bathwater—soak for twenty minutes. Apply shampoo to pre-wetted hair and massage well.

● *Side effects:* Sensitivity reactions rare.

● *Special advantages:* Bland skin cleaner, removes skin debris in psoriasis, dandruff, eczema.

▲ Ionil T

(Coal tar and salicylic acid with benzalkonium.)

● *Basic precautions:* For external use only.

● *Proper usage:* Shampoo to be used daily, if necessary.

● *Side effects:* Sensitivity reactions.

SELENIUM SULPHIDE

Selenium sulphide (F)

(Commercially made into a suspension cream containing 2.5 per cent selenium sulphide.)

▲ Lenium shampoo

● *Basic precautions:* Do not use on broken or denuded skin or if hair is going to receive a permanent wave shortly. Do not use within two days of tinting hair. Keep clear of eyes. May discolour metals. Wash hands thoroughly and scrub fingernails after use.

● *Proper usage:* Shampoo twice weekly for two weeks, then once weekly for two weeks, then every three to six weeks. Sometimes Lenium encourages hair to become greasy, if so use non-medicated shampoo as necessary.

● *Side effects:* Sensitivity reactions are rare.

● *Special advantages:* Effective medical control of dandruff, scaly conditions of scalp.

▲ Selsun shampoo
- *Basic precautions:* Thoroughly wash off other medication. Do not use in conjunction with metal hair clips or decoration, before or after hair tinting, or if scalp has any sore places or abrasions. Wash hands after use and scrub nails.
- *Proper usage:* First wash hair with soap or soap shampoo (not detergent shampoo). Apply Selsun to wet scalp and work up lather—keep in contact with scalp for three minutes and then thoroughly rinse, repeat and then wash hands. Repeat twice weekly for two weeks, then weekly for two weeks and then occasionally if necessary.
- *Special advantages:* As for Lenium.

SOAP AND SPIRIT
▲ Soft soap and Spirit soap
(General all-purpose skin cleansers using soap, in its traditional sense, for a local antiseptic.)

ANTISEPTICS FOR PREVENTING INFECTION OR SPREAD OF INFECTION

BENZALKONIUM
▲ Capitol, Drapolene, Roccal
- *Proper usage:* Little used outside hospital and clinic practice, although they are excellent non-irritant wound cleansers and antiseptics. Dilution has to be made accurately, however, for specific uses.
- *Side effects:* None, if properly diluted.
- *Special advantages:* They maintain a high reputation in medicine, due to extreme stability and compatibility with many other substances. But apart from Drapolene, a particularly useful remedy in urinary ammonia dermatitis (nappy rash), little used as prescription or OTC remedies.

CETRIMIDE
(*See* skin cleaners and shampoos in previous section.)
▲ Cetavlex, Morsep, Propa PH, Savlon cream and Cetrimide cream (F)
- *Proper usage:* As for cetrimide.
- *Side effects:* As for cetrimide.
- *Special advantages:* Useful, non-irritating creams for minor wounds and abrasions.

CHLORHEXIDINE
▲ Acriflex
(General-purpose antiseptic cream.)
- *Proper usage:* Apply twice daily.
- *Side effects:* Sensitivity reactions occur rarely.
▲ Hibiscrub, Hibisol
(Mainly used as surgical 'scrub up' preparations. *See* benzalkonium, above.)
▲ Hibitane
(Mainly used in hospital and clinical practice.)

▲ PHiso-Med, PHiso-Hex

- *Basic precautions:* Should always be washed off afterwards when used as a cleansing agent.
- *Proper usage:* Apply to wet hands, body or scalp. Rinse well afterwards.
- *Side effects:* Sensitivity reactions are rare.
- *Special advantages:* Efficient for skin cleaning, especially around spots and boils.

▲ Rotersept

(A useful nipple and breast antiseptic.)

- *Basic precautions:* As it is an aerosol preparation, read instructions carefully.
- *Proper usage:* Use before and after feeding baby. Spray at a two-inch range, giving brief burst of spray. Will stain in contact with chlorides (body fluids/salt).
- *Side effects:* Sensitivity reactions are rare.
- *Special advantages:* Greatly reduces risk of inflammation of breast (mastitis) and cracked nipples.

CHLORINATED LIME

▲ Chlorinated lime solution (F)

(An old-fashioned but effective mild antiseptic. Little used today.)

Eusol

- *Proper usage:* Used as an antiseptic wound and cleaning agent. Apply on gauze and place on wound or ulcer.
- *Special advantages:* Widely used for cleaning varicose ulcers, bed sores and operational wounds.

CHLOROXYLENOL

▲ Chloroxylenol solution (F)
▲ Dettol

(Useful general-purpose skin antiseptics.)

- *Special advantages:* A quick-acting skin antiseptic which, unlike many skin antiseptics, works well in the presence of soaps.

HEXACHLOROPHANE

▲ Hexachlorophane dusting powder, Ster-Zac powder

- *Basic precautions:* Do not use on children under age of two. Do not apply to damaged skin.
- *Side effects:* Sensitivity reactions are rare.
- *Special advantages:* Useful for treating furunculosis (multiple septic spots and boils).

HYDROGEN PEROXIDE

(Relatively weak germicide which is not used a great deal now.)

▲ Hydrogen peroxide solution, Hioxyl

(Cream containing hydrogen peroxide used for leg ulcers and skin cleaning.)

POVIDONE-IODINE

(Iodine in the form of a tincture or solution is an extremely powerful and safe, but unfashionable antiseptic.)

▲ Betadine

- *Proper usage:* A wide range of Betadine preparations are available. These contain iodine in combination with a substance that liberates iodine in solutions, and are thus applicable to those open wounds and abrasions where iodine would once have been used.

● *Side effects:* Sensitivity reactions are rare.

● *Special advantages:* This method of the liberation of the iodine minimises the pain that usually follows the use of iodine, which has led to the latter's unfashionability as a disinfectant. These prescriptions are relatively expensive, however, and are said to be no more effective than cetrimide preparations.

▲ **Disphex**

▲ **Disadine**
● *Proper usage:* As Betadine.
● *Side effects:* As Betadine.
● *Special advantages:* This is a dry spray powder used for bedsores and varicose ulcers, it is a useful, non-messy preparation.

Skin infections and their treatment

Sometimes the skin becomes infected, and common examples of infection include impetigo, boils, spots and fungus infections (athlete's foot and tinea). Although there are a great many remedies used to combat skin infection, in many cases all that is really necessary is suitable hygiene and the removal of infected debris from the skin. There is a constant danger in using antibiotics or antibacterial drugs locally on the skin that general sensitivity to these compounds may result or strains of germs which are resistant to antibiotics may develop. This may limit the use of that drug in a subsequent general or serious illness. Even some 'skin-only' antibiotics (eg neomycin) can cause sensitivity reactions. Some special 'skin' uses—ie around the eye and ear—are described in the chapter on the eye and ear.

GENERAL SKIN INFECTION REMEDIES

DIBROMOPROPAMIDINE

▲ **Brulidine cream**
● *Proper usage:* After cleaning the graze or burn, cream should be spread on sterile dressing and applied to skin.
● *Side effects:* Sensitivity reactions are rare.
● *Special advantages:* An economical antiseptic cream with a wide range of activity against many skin bacteria. Will also kill many skin fungi, including those causing ringworm and athlete's foot.

FRAMYCETIN

Framygen
● *Proper usage:* Apply directly to infected skin thrice daily.
● *Side effects:* Sensitivity reactions are rare.
● *Special advantages:* Few side effects. Effective in most skin infections including barber's rash and impetigo.

Sofra-Tulle
(Squares of sterile lightweight non-stick (lanoline) gauze)
- *Basic precautions:* In order to retain sterile nature of dressing, remove each piece with sterile tweezers or needle.
- *Proper usage:* Apply once daily.
- *Side effects:* Rare sensitivity to framycetin; more common sensitivity to lanolin.
- *Special advantages:* Wide range of action against bacteria. As a non-stick dressing it is useful for infected burns and ulcers.

FUSIDIC ACID
Fucidin (ointment, cream, gel or gauze)
- *Basic precautions:* Keep away from eyes.
- *Proper usage:* Apply ointment or gel four times daily, gauze once daily.
- *Side effects:* Sensitivity reactions are rare.
- *Special advantages:* Very effective against problems caused by staphylococcus (boils, carbuncles, impetigo, infected eczema). Can penetrate normal skin (that has not been cut or grazed) and so can reach infection under skin.

GENTAMICIN
Cidomycin, Genticin
- *Proper usage:* Apply four times daily and cover with dressing.
- *Side effects:* Sensitivity reactions.
- *Special advantages:* Both have a very wide spectrum of antiseptic activity. Useful in all primary and secondary infections of skin.

NEOMYCIN
Myciguent and Neomycin cream (F)
- *Basic precautions:* Do not apply to infected eczema.
- *Proper usage:* Apply four times daily.
- *Side effects:* Sensitivity reactions are rare.
- *Special advantages:* Broad action against many bacterial infected skin conditions; also prevents the action of some secondary infecting germs.

NITROFURAZONE
Furacin
- *Proper usage:* Apply twice daily.
- *Side effects:* Sensitivity reactions.
- *Special advantages:* A good general skin antiseptic.

POLYNOXYLIN
▲ Anaflex, Ponoxylan (multiple preparations)
- *Proper usage:* Once or twice daily.
- *Special advantages:* Effective against wide range of bacteria and fungi. Is particularly effective in 'damp' or 'wet' skin areas and so is useful in nappy rash or for use on the sexual skin or around anus.

PROPAMIDINE
▲ M & B antiseptic cream
- *Proper usage:* Apply to cleaned skin twice daily—avoid prolonged use.
- *Side effects:* Very rare.
- *Special advantages:* A powerful bacteriocidal agent with wide range of action.

TETRACYCLINE
Achromycin
(Also used widely for treatment of eye infections. *See* Chapter 13, page 137.)
- *Basic precautions:* Tetracycline is a widely used and effective antibiotic which is often prescribed for oral use. It is also effective when applied on the skin. This means that the possibility of skin-induced allergy to the drug is sometimes overlooked.
- *Proper usage:* Apply three times a day.
- *Side effects:* Rare, but preparations contain lanoline which is often implicated in sensitivity reactions.
- *Special advantages:* Very effective broad-spectrum antibiotic product.

TRICLOCARBAN
▲ Cutisan (multiple preparations)
- *Proper usage:* Apply to the infected area and the skin beyond it.
- *Special advantages:* A mild antiseptic useful for infected eczema and infected contact dermatitis. Also used for acne.

FUNGUS INFECTION REMEDIES

Wise physicians like to identify the particular fungus causing an infection because some infections are best treated by a specific fungus antibiotic. To identify the various fungal infections that produce ringworm and athlete's foot a microscope is necessary. In the past many products like phenol, potassium permanganate and various dyes were used for treatment. Most of these have been discarded as better and safer remedies have evolved.

Preparations commonly used

BENZOIC ACID
▲ Whitfield's ointment
- *Basic precautions:* Do not apply if skin is inflamed (red or sore) around the fungus infection. In such cases allow inflammation to settle or get advice about a suitable skin antiseptic. Then apply ointment twice daily.
- *Proper usage:* Apply and continue for five days after skin appears to have returned to normal.
- *Side effects:* Inflammation is exacerbated if applied to already inflamed skin.
- *Special advantages:* A cheap remedy that works particularly well on hard skin (as on the sole of the foot).

AMPHOTERICIN
Fungilin
- *Proper usage:* Apply four times daily; do not rub in.
- *Special advantages:* A specific remedy for fungal infections caused by *candida albicans* (thrush). Useful for napkin rash where thrush is implicated.

CHLORPHENESIN
▲ Mycil and Chlorphenesin cream and powder (F)
- *Proper usage:* First wash skin area and dry with a towel specially kept for this

purpose. Rub in ointment or cream twice daily and dust surrounding skin with powder. Shake powder into socks and shoes before wearing. Continue treatment for a week after skin appears normal.

● *Side effects:* Sensitivity reactions are rare.

● *Special advantages:* Is both antiseptic and antifungal, especially to *tinea pedis* (athlete's foot), *tinea cruris* and prickly heat.

CLOTRIMAZOLE

▲ Canesten cream and spray
Canesten powder

● *Basic precautions:* Causes mild burning or irritation on rare occasions. Keep spray away from eyes and mucous surfaces and flames; do not inhale.

● *Proper usage:* Wash and dry skin. Rub in gently thrice daily for one month and then for two weeks after infection disappears. The spray should be used in the same manner as cream. The powder should be dusted around area and used in socks and footwear.

● *Special advantages:* A broad-spectrum antifungal that is effective in all fungus infections. Prolonged use after treatment is necessary if relapses are to be avoided.

ECONAZOLE

Ecostatin, Pevaryl and Econazole nitrate cream (F)

● *Basic precautions:* Do not use near eyes.

● *Proper usage:* Massage preparation in night and morning. Continue for six days after cure.

● *Side effects:* Irritation and redness of skin follows use on rare occasions.

● *Special advantages:* Wide-acting, broad-spectrum antifungal which is effective against all known fungi, moulds and yeasts.

MICONAZOLE

▲ Daktarin, Dermonistat and Miconazole nitrate (F)
Brentan cream

● *Proper usage:* For skin—apply ointments twice daily and for ten days after cure. Apply powder around treated skin. For nails—apply daily and cover with waterproof (occlusive) dressing. Continue until new nail has grown.

● *Side effects:* Sensitivity reactions are rare.

● *Special advantages:* A good general fungicide that also has bacteria-killing properties. Useful for fungus nail problems.

NATAMYCIN

Pimafucin

● *Proper usage:* For skin—apply thrice daily and for one week after cure. For nails—apply similarly for three months.

● *Special advantages:* An antithrush preparation suitable for mucous membranes (mouth, around genitalia and anus). Used for nail infections, if due to thrush.

NYSTATIN

Nystan

● *Proper usage:* Apply powder, cream, gel or ointment four times daily and for one week after cure has been effected.

● *Special advantages:* A very well-tolerated, broad-spectrum antifungal with no side effects.

PECILOCIN
Variotin
● *Basic precautions:* Do not apply to inflamed skin or to eczematous or infected skin.
● *Proper usage:* Apply thrice daily.
● *Side effects:* Sensitivity reactions are rare.
● *Special advantages:* A specific tinea remedy which is not inhibited by skin grease (fungus infections of foot, groin or scalp).

TOLNAFTATE
▲ Tinaderm
● *Proper usage:* Massage ointment in twice daily. Use powder around infection.
● *Side effects:* Rare hypersensitivity, redness, itching.
● *Special advantages:* Wide-spectrum antifungal remedy (not effective against thrush). Quick-acting, non-irritant even to inflamed areas. Effective in areas where perspiration is a problem.

UNDECENOATE
▲ Tineafax, Mycota, Monphytal
● *Proper usage:* Apply night and morning after washing and drying skin. Rub well in, paint or powder on and around infected skin. Keep feet as dry as possible. Change socks daily.
● *Special advantages:* A very well-tolerated specific remedy for athlete's foot.

Skin protection and skin camouflage

Sunlight is, potentially, the worst skin-damaging hazard, and every year many thousands of sunburn cases occur, some of which are bad enough to be admitted to hospital. A tan is falsely equated with a healthy look and is in all probability a psychological hangover from the days when paleness meant anaemia, tuberculosis and rickets. We now know that poor diet was related to the first two evils. Lack of sunlight contributed to the occurrence of rickets, as the skin manufactures vitamin D, which is necessary for the prevention of rickets, only if there is adequate exposure to sunlight. Regular exposure to daylight rather than sunbathing is all that is necessary to prevent rickets in non-coloured races, and today's fashionable tan is purely a cosmetic preference.

Because of the hazards of sunburn, quite effective sun-screening compounds have been developed. These filter out the very short wavelengths of light that are associated with skin-burning and yet allow the longer wavelengths to encourage the skin to react (protectively) to prevent skin damage. Nevertheless, all sun-screeners delay tanning. Ultraviolet light exposure not only tans the skin, but it accelerates skin-ageing by encouragement of fragmentation of the skin's elastic tissues. Prolonged exposure to a high dosage of ultraviolet light predisposes one to the development of skin cancer. Certain drugs can be 'photosensitisers'—in other words make the individual extra-sensitive to sunlight. Certain of the tetracycline drugs have this unfortunate propensity. (You can refer to the various basic precautions and side effect sections for more information on tetracycline.) Certain diseases also produce secondary photosensitivity, especially porphyria, and so does the handling of certain plants (eg grasses, primulas and so on).

Secondary to sun-induced skin damage, skin problems are brought about by exposure to chemical skin irritants and also by exposure to that most universal of all skin irritants—water. To some extent the so-called 'barrier creams' give protection against both hazards. Mankind has been using oil and grease as a skin protective since the beginning of time, and more recently silicones have been incorporated into barrier creams in an attempt to improve on the more traditional remedies. Water damages the skin in a curious way—by making it lose its 'waterproof' quality. Once this occurs tissue fluids tend to escape from the subcutaneous tissues and noxious substances and invading organisms gain easy access to the deeper unprotected areas of skin. Skin protection against water is necessary sometimes in the case of incontinence, nappy rashes and 'ostomy' routines.

Camouflaging preparations can do a lot to mask certain irremedial skin abnormalities—for example facial 'port wine stains' and scarred areas.

SUN-SCREENER PROTECTION

AMINOBENZOIC ACID
▲ Aminobenzoic acid lotion (F)
- *Proper usage:* Apply undiluted and allow to dry before exposure to sun. Repeat every two hours and after bathing.
- *Special advantages:* A good short-return preparation.

MEXENONE
▲ Uvistat, Uvistat L and Mexenone cream (F)
- *Proper usage:* Apply liberally and rub in twice daily. Repeat if skin becomes wet through sweating or bathing.
- *Special advantages:* Long-acting, can be used on scalp; special lip-salve preparation for winter use.

PADIMATE
▲ Spectraban
- *Basic precautions:* Avoid applying near eyes and in the presence of a naked flame.
- *Proper usage:* Apply evenly and liberally to all exposed areas once daily—repeat after swimming or heavy sweating.
- *Side effects:* Sensitivity reactions are rare.
- *Special advantages:* A single daily application still gives considerable protection after sweat-producing exercise (75 per cent); after swimming it is 50 per cent. However, it must be applied forty-five minutes before exposure. Does not rub off on clothing. Useful in preventing secondary photosensitivity.

SKIN-IRRITANT PROTECTION AND OVER-HYDRATION REMEDIES

ZINC AND OIL PREPARATIONS
▲ Morhulin, Vasogen and Zinc formulary preparations (F), Oily cream (F), Paraffin ointment (F) and Hydrous wool fat (F)

▲ Vaseline

- *Proper usage:* Apply all preparations liberally before exposure. Rub in well.
- *Side effects:* Sensitivity.
- *Special advantages:* Economical and, according to some authorities, as good as more expensive products. Vasogen contains added (waterproofing) silicone. A bland, safe type of preparation for skin, packaged as a 'baby cream'.

DIMETHICONE

▲ Siopel and Dimethicone cream (F)

- *Basic precautions:* Do not apply to inflamed or 'weeping' skin.
- *Proper usage:* Apply liberally and rub in well three to five times daily before exposure for five days. After that apply twice daily.
- *Side effects:* Sensitivity reactions are rare.
- *Special advantages:* Contains water-repellent silicones.

Sprilon

Specialised use for incontinence or 'ostomy' care. May be used also in nappy rashes and bedsores. See manufacturer's instructions.

MULTI-FORMULATION REMEDIES

▲ Dust barrier cream (F), Water-repellent barrier (F), Oil-repellent barrier (F), Paraffin-type oil-repellent (F), Kaolin/Soap skin conditioning cream (F)

- *Proper usage:* Apply to clean, dry hands sparingly to whole hand not omitting backs of hands and sides of fingers, nail folds and under nails. To obtain best results apply twice daily for ten days before exposure. Then apply once daily before exposure. Use skin conditioner cream after using barrier.

▲ Natuderm

- *Proper usage:* Apply thinly three times daily before or immediately after exposure to harmful factors. Rub in gently.
- *Side effects:* Sensitivity reactions are rare.
- *Special advantages:* Has a fat content closely matched to that of human skin grease—replaces artificially depleted skin protection.

SKIN CAMOUFLAGE

▲ Boots covering cream, Covermark

These preparations are for special conditions. They are usually supplied initially by a hospital department where an expert will provide full information on their use.

Anti-itch (antipruritic) preparations

For many years local anaesthetics and locally applied antihistamines were widely used to provide antipruritic treatment. These were generally multi-formulation remedies. In recent times it has become general practice to eschew such preparations because of the risk of sensitisation which could exacerbate symptoms. Many antihistamines taken by mouth are, however, very effective as antipruritics.

General note: Many widely advertised OTC preparations contain local anaesthetics.

Usually it takes fairly prolonged usage before allergic manifestations occur. But unfortunately should such side effects develop, symptoms may be confused with a relapse of the original complaint—ie itching. The following three anaesthetic-containing preparations is a far from comprehensive list, but readers can spot the presence of local anaesthetics in other preparations by recognising the names of compounds commonly used in this way.

Examples of antipruritic preparations containing anaesthetics

Proprietary preparation	Anaesthetic
▲ Lanacane	Benzocaine
▲ Locan	Amylocaine, amethocaine
▲ Dermidex	Lidocaine

ANTIPRURITIC DRUGS COMMONLY USED

The preparations listed below are all topical applications except for trimeprazine.

Active principal	Proprietary preparation	Formulary preparation
Zinc	▲ Caladryl	▲ Calamine application
	▲ Dermogesic	▲ Calamine cream
		lotion
		oily
		ointment
Crotamiton	▲ Eurax ointment and lotion	
Trimeprazine	Vallergan tablets and syrups	Trimeprazine tartrate

ZINC PREPARATIONS
▲ Caladryl
Probably best *not* used, as it contains an antihistamine.

▲ Dermogesic
Probably best *not* used, as it contains a local anaesthetic.

▲ Calamine products:
Calamine application (F), cream (F), lotion (F), ointment (F)
General note: Calamine preparations are effective probably because of their mild zinc content. Local zinc salts are mildly astringent and antiseptic. The various formulary preparations are used fairly arbitrarily according to local circumstances, eg the lotion is more astringent than the cream and is therefore applied to stings and bites. Creams, ointments and oily lotions are used if drying or cracking of the skin is best prevented.
● *Proper usage:* Apply as required.

CROTAMITON
(A dual-purpose remedy for itching and scabies (a disease that has itching as a common symptom).)
▲ Eurax
● *Basic precautions:* Avoid using on oozing rashes and around eyes.
● *Proper usage:* For itching—massage in twice daily. For scabies—use after a soapy

bath and drying. Apply to body from chin to feet, rubbing well in areas between fingers, wrists, inner and outer aspects of elbows, under arms, below breasts, in umbilicus, buttocks and thighs. Allow to dry. Re-apply in twenty-four hours; then after a further twenty-four hours bath thoroughly. Change clothes and send bed linen to laundry.

● *Special advantages:* Useful in diseases like scabies which are often misdiagnosed. It can thus be used on an itchy rash which will not clear.

TRIMEPRAZINE
Vallergan and Trimeprazine tartrate (F)

● *Basic precautions:* Avoid alcoholic drinks while using this preparation.
● *Proper dosage:* Composition and strength—tablets 10 mg; syrup 7.5 mg to every 5 ml; forte syrup 30 mg to every 5 ml. Adults: 10 mg three to four times daily. Children: 2.5–5 mg three to four times daily.
● *Side effects:* Generally drowsiness; sometimes disturbing dreams, dryness of mouth, nasal stuffiness, headache, disturbance of mood. Rarely skin rashes.
● *Special advantages:* A useful adjunct to local treatment for skin problems complicated by severe itching.

Acne medication

In almost no other skin disease are the various factors that affect the condition of the skin more clearly demonstrated as in acne. It is a curious and infuriating skin condition. Most skin disease responds adversely to stress, emotion and upset. Acne is made very much worse if such factors are present. Many diseases are improved by sunshine—acne is certainly better during the summer months. The skin is very sensitive to hormones—especially the sex hormones. In acne the increased greasiness of the skin (or more accurately changes in the stickiness of the skin grease brought about by certain hormones) is closely related to hormone changes in adolescence and early adult life.

Acne sufferers quite often become obsessed by skin cleaning when spots spoil the look of their skin. This is understandable but it is important to realise that germs and infection are not primarily the cause of the acne spot and mini-abscess that usually forms around it. Due to hormone swings and changes, the grease-secreting glands become overblown with thick skin grease (sebum). This sebum cannot escape to the skin's surface to carry out its usual lubricating function. Sometimes the glands become so distended that they rupture subcutaneously into the skin where the grease reacts within the subcutaneous tissues to form a mini-abscess. This is essentially a sterile 'foreign body' type of reaction, although in some cases skin germs will complicate the picture and acne becomes infected. Acne is treated in various ways, but as far as local prescription and OTC remedies are concerned these evolve around skin peeling agents, skin abrasives and bacterial control. Sometimes very limited application of steroid-containing remedies is justified. In severe acne the antibiotic tetracycline is often taken by mouth and some women are prescribed certain contraceptive pill-type treatments to alleviate acne.

LOCAL PREPARATIONS FOR ACNE

SALICYLIC ACID

▲ Avrogel, Dermaclean, DDD lotion
▲ Salicylic acid and sulphur cream

- *Proper usage, side effects:* Salicylic acid dissolves keratin (the horny protein of the skin) and so the skin tends to soften, swell and subsequently scale. A trial and error method of use is necessary for these remedies. The aim is to soften the skin around the grease glands so that sebum is discharged and the mini-abscesses of acne are not allowed to form. Application of too little of the preparation will have no effect. Too much will produce a dry and sore skin. Nightly application, washed off carefully next day, for two or three weeks will demonstrate whether or not acne is improving.

SULPHUR (WITH OR WITHOUT RESORCINOL)

RESORCINOL

General note: Certain organisms on the skin convert sulphur (a relatively inert substance when used locally) into a compound that limits the growth of certain skin bacteria without actually killing them. Thus it is said to be bacteriostatic, not bacteriocidal. The effectiveness of sulphur on infected skin conditions is presumably because it does not alter the skin's ecology too much (many skin bacteria are protective) and yet controls heavy infection. It also has a keratin-softening property and thus prevents acne and mini-abscess production.

Resorcinol is mildly bacteriocidal and fungicidal. It has the facility of penetrating the intact skin and working slowly to kill deep infection. It is, therefore, also effective in controlling the mini-abscess infection of acne. These various actions provide the popularity of these compounds for acne treatment and control.

▲ Acnil
▲ Clearasil

- *Basic precautions:* Do not use in cases of *acne rosacea*—a chronic skin condition characterised by redness and pustules on the face. Resorcinol preparations should not be used by persons with thyroid deficiency (myxoedema). Keep away from eyes.
- *Proper usage:* Apply preparations twice daily until the acne clears.
- *Side effects:* Sensitivity reactions are rare.

▲ Dome-Acne cream, lotion, Dome-Acne medicated cleanser

- *Basic precautions:* Shake liquids well to dispense particles.
- *Proper usage:* In severe cases the skin should be cleansed with a moistened sponge using Dome-Acne Medicated. In less severe cases apply twice daily after ordinary washing.
- *Side effects:* As for formulary preparations.

Eskamel

- *Basic precautions:* Avoid using on acutely inflamed areas of skin.
- *Proper usage:* Wash skin with soap and water. Apply to skin thinly (do not rub in) once a day or twice if skin is very oily.
- *Side effects:* Excessive redness or scaling may occur in which case stop treatment

for a few days and recommence with smaller amounts used at less frequent intervals.
- *Special advantages:* Can be applied under cosmetics.

▲ **pHiso-Ac, Wigglesworth acne cream**
▲ **Formulary sulphur (F), zinc (F), resorcinol preparations (F)**
- *Proper usage:* Apply to washed face daily. In general, follow advice as for Eskamel or manufacturer's instructions.
- *Side effects:* Occasional sensitivity.

BENZOYL PEROXIDE

▲ **Acetoxyl, Acnegel, Benoxyl, Panoxyl, Quinoderm,* Vanair**
- *Basic precautions:* Keep away from mouth, eyes, and use cautiously on neck. May bleach clothing and fabric.
- *Proper usage:* Wash face and then apply product. Apply once daily—a mild burning sensation is to be expected and a moderate peeling will occur in most cases. If this is excessive stop treatment until it settles, then recommence treatment.
- *Side effects:* Occasionally extreme redness. Stop therapy and consult doctor.
- *Special advantages:* Benzoyl peroxide is claimed to be specifically antibacterial against an organism commonly present in acne follicles (*corynebacterium acnes*). These proprietary preparations are available in various strengths. Some are also marketed with an added sulphur content and these have the therapeutic advantages of sulphur (*see* General note, opposite page).

*Quinoderm contains potassium hydroquinoline which has antibacterial, antifungal and deodorant properties.

ALUMINIUM

▲ **Brasivol**
(An abrasive powder in a soap-detergent base.)
- *Basic precautions:* Do not use if face appears to have obvious superficial skin veins. Do not use close to eyes or mouth. If electric razor is being used shave before using Brasivol.
- *Proper usage:* Brasivol is manufactured in three grades (fine, medium and coarse). Usually start with *fine* grade product. It should be used to clear face by rubbing gently over the wetted face with a circular motion thrice daily and then thoroughly rinsed off. If no response is obvious after three weeks, *medium* grade should be used. The *coarse* grade preparation should be reserved for longer-term maintenance after suitable response has been obtained.
- *Side effects:* Over-enthusiastic use can cause inflammation of face.
- *Special advantages:* A mechanical rather than chemical action removes grease and prevents acne spots developing (surgical dermabrasion is a traumatic but effective treatment in cases of severe acne).

POLYETHYLENE

▲ **Ionax Scrub**
General note: This preparation is really a soap substitute. The polyethylene it contains protects the underlying skin from air and thus tends to prevent the opening of the sebaceous gland developing into a blackhead and then into an acne mini-abscess.

- *Basic precautions:* Wet face thoroughly before use.
- *Proper usage:* Use as soap thrice daily to clean skin.
- *Side effects:* None.
- *Special advantages:* Very bland treatment for sensitive skins.

TRETINOIN
Retin-A

- *Basic precautions:* Do not use with any other skin treatment, especially peeling agents. Avoid exposure to strong sunlight and ultraviolet light. Do not use after sunburn or if skin is repeatedly exposed to extremes of wind and cold. Keep away from eyes and mouth, cuts or abrasions. Do not use if eczema or dermatitis occur.
- *Proper usage:* Apply once or twice daily *only* to skin area where acne spots occur. Only apply enough to moisten skin over spot. Excessive application does not produce more effective response which, in any case, is very slow (in six to eight weeks). Once response is obtained a less frequent use is sufficient to maintain clear skin.
- *Side effects:* Over-use causes severe redness, irritation and discomfort. Increased or decreased skin colouring may occur.
- *Special advantages:* None.

STEROID WITH ANTIBIOTIC TREATMENT
General note: Steroid use on the skin is covered elsewhere in a general way (page 96). There is some justification for short-term use of steroid antibiotic preparation in severe and resistant acne. This should not be continued for more than three weeks.

Actinac

- *Basic precautions:* Not suitable if patient is sensitive to chloramphenicol, butoxyethyl nicotinate, allantoin or sulphur. Do not use during pregnancy. Avoid contact with eyes or mouth.
- *Proper usage:* To be applied with cotton wool at night and in the morning for four days initially. After that at night only. Continue for three nights after suitable response has been obtained.
- *Side effects:* Redness of skin.
- *Special advantages:* Helpful in severe intractable acne, and as a standby treatment for acne flare-ups.

Neo-Medrone

- *Basic precautions:* Do not use if sensitive to sulphur, neomycin, aluminium.
- *Proper usage:* As for Actinac.
- *Side effects:* As for Actinac.
- *Special advantages:* As for Actinac.

Medrone Acne Lotion

General note: This preparation relies on the relatively weak antibacterial action of sulphur to protect the skin from the possibility of a flare-up of infection caused by the steroid it contains. In practice, problems seldom occur, but the manufacturer recommends using Neo-Medrone if infection is present. In acne *per se* infection is almost always present (*see* Neo-Medrone).

Quinoderm Cream with hydrocortisone

General note: This preparation contains potassium hydroxyquinoline as a bacteriocide instead of an antibiotic.

- *Basic precautions:* Avoid use during pregnancy.
- *Proper usage:* Spread thinly and massage into skin thrice daily, covering the whole area of acne, not just individual spots.
- *Side effects:* None, other than those occasioned by long-term abuse (*see* steroid preparations, page 96).
- *Special advantages:* Lack of side effects—also effective in other skin conditions with an infective element, eg impetigo and shaving rash.

MIXED INGREDIENTS

▲ Biactol, Clean & Clear, Germolene, Sevilan, Spotaway, Swiss Biofacial, TCP, Torbetol, Valderma

General note: These proprietary products are widely used. Patients may suffer from the sum of their ingredients as far as side effects are concerned and benefit from the sum total of their therapeutic action. Generally speaking, they have no advantages over the simpler products detailed in previous sections.

SYSTEMIC (SWALLOWED) REMEDIES FOR ACNE

Tetracyclines are the commonest drugs used. *See* Chapter 4, page 61.

Warts, corns and calluses

Corns and calluses are brought about by the pressure exerted by shoe fitting and the slip between shoe and foot. They are unknown among peoples who constantly remain barefoot and they disappear during long periods of bed-rest. Treatment, therefore, should be directed toward footwear rather than medicaments, although salicylic acid is often applied and is the active ingredient in most corn plasters. Warts are caused by a virus. Most treatments for warts endeavour to produce a chemical burn and thus destroy the wart or to kill its virus content. In many cases warts are multiple and there is no doubt that one wart usually leads to a small colony developing. Like many tumours, warts manufacture a substance that tends to prevent the body getting rid of them, and this allows the development of 'satellite' warts. If one directs treatment initially to the largest and most mature warts, these will wither and the wart defence substance will diminish rapidly; in this fashion the body often quickly rids itself of satellite, or offspring warts. Warts seem to have a fairly stable natural history if left alone and the body gradually develops antibodies against the virus. When this reaches an effective level warts disappear. The popularity of folklore charms and cures for warts which claimed to 'cure warts overnight' was based on the fact that they were about to regress anyway.

Preparations commonly used

Active principal	Proprietary preparation	Formulary preparation
Podophyllum	▲ Posalfilin	▲ Podophyllum Paint

Table continued on next page

Table continued from previous page

Active principal	Proprietary preparation	Formulary preparation
Salicylic acid	▲ Avrogel ▲ Ayrton's corn and wart paint ▲ Compound W ▲ Duofilm ▲ Salactol ▲ Verrugon ▲ Wartex	▲ Salicylic Acid Collodion
Acetic acid	▲ Cupal Wart Solvent	▲ Glacial acetic acid
Benzalkonium	▲ Callusolve	
Formaldehyde	▲ Veracur	
Glutaraldehyde	▲ Glutarol	

PODOPHYLLUM

▲ Posalfilin and Podophyllum paint (F)

- *Basic precautions:* Do not apply to healthy skin or near eyes or mucous surfaces.
- *Proper usage:* Place felt corn ring around wart (not a corn plaster) allowing wart to show through the hole. Apply minimal amount to cover wart and cover with waterproof plaster. Reapply thrice weekly. When wart is soft and spongy cover with dry dressing only. If wart does not fall off in a day or two repeat procedure.
- *Side effects:* Chemical burns or dermatitis may be caused if too much is used.

SALICYLIC ACID

▲ Avrogel, Ayrton's, Duofilm, Verrugon, Wartex
▲ Compound W, Salactol and Salicylic acid (F)

- *Basic precautions:* Do not apply to healthy skin, near eyes or mucous surfaces.
- *Proper usage:* Paint wart, allow to dry being careful not to allow paint to 'run'. Cover with waterproof dressing. After one day remove dressing and rub surface of wart with pumice stone until it is smooth. Repeat. When wart starts to fade relinquish treatment. If wart is still growing after one week repeat treatment.
- *Side effects:* As for podophyllum.

ACETIC ACID

▲ Cupal
▲ Glacial acetic acid

- *Basic precautions:* Apply with orange stick.
- *Proper usage:* As for salicylic acid.

BENZALKONIUM

▲ Callusolve

Details as for acetic acid.

FORMALDEHYDE

▲ Veracur

Details as for acetic acid.

GLUTARALDEHYDE
▲ Glutarol
Details as for acetic acid.

Eczema and psoriasis treatments

Although these two conditions often look very different, their treatment merges and overlaps. Dermatitis and eczema appear to be closely related diseases, the term 'dermatitis' being applied when the skin is reacting acutely with secretion and soreness; eczema describes a dry, itchy, scaly condition. Psoriasis is also a disease characterised by skin scaling. Its basic cause is still unknown. The management of both of these conditions demands a high measure of collaboration between doctor and patient. Treatment is quite frequently ineffective and has to be changed. Skin cleaning and conditioning is often necessary and the remedies described under *Skin cleaners and shampoos* are effective. Sometimes antihistamines can be useful, as also anti-itch preparations. For information on the former, *see* Chapter 12, pages 132–133, and Chapter 14, pages 148–149, while general information on the latter drugs (among them Vallergan) can be found on pages 87–89. Skin irritant and hydration remedies and anti-infective remedies may also be indicated (*see* page 79). There are, however, a few specific treatments for psoriasis and eczema; preparations containing corticosteroids are particularly useful—although they are frequently abused.

Coal tar preparations hold an important place in the treatment of eczema and psoriasis. *Ichthammol* has a milder action and is useful in less acute problems. *Urea* is a hydrating agent (prevents dehydration) and tends to enhance the efficacy of other drugs. *Dithranol* is specially helpful in some cases of psoriasis. These basic drugs are often combined with other substances to produce a bewildering combination of pastes, ointments and creams.

Local steroid preparations can be classified as weak, moderately potent, potent and very potent. With increased potency comes an increase of side effects. As such substances are in no way curative, the lowest potency that will alleviate the condition should be the chosen preparation. To further complicate the picture, other drugs, including antibiotics, are often prescribed for use with the local steroid creams and ointments. There is little evidence that this method of treatment, though popular, has validity in the long-term management of eczema and psoriasis.

SPECIFIC NON-STEROID TREATMENTS

COAL TAR PREPARATIONS
▲ Carbo-Dome, Coltapaste, Psoriderm, Tarband, Calamine and coal tar (F), Coal tar and salicylic ointment (F), Coal tar paste and paint (F), Zinc and coal tar paste (F) and Zinc paste coal tar bandage (F)

- *Basic precautions:* Do not apply near eyes or mucous surfaces; do not use if suffering from acute attacks of eczema.
- *Proper usage:* Apply two to four times daily.
- *Side effects:* Sensitivity reactions are rare.
- *Special advantages:* Effective preparations with very few side effects.

ICHTHAMMOL PREPARATIONS

▲ **Ichthopaste, Icthaband, Ichthammol ointment (F), Zinc paste (F), Ichthammol bandage (F)**
Details: As for coal tar preparations.

UREA PREPARATIONS

▲ **Aquadrate, Calmurid**
Details: As for coal tar preparations. Urea products are more suitable for children.
- *Special advantages:* Can be used for acute eczemas.

DITHRANOL PREPARATIONS

Psoradrate

▲ **Dithrocream, Dithrolan, Stie-Lasan, Exolan and Dithranol ointment and paste (F)**
Dithranol ointment and paste
- *Basic precautions:* These apply generally for treatment of psoriasis. Sensitivity may sometimes occur in which case do not use. Do not use on acute forms of psoriasis. May stain clothing. Keep away from eyes.
- *Proper usage:* Apply sparingly at night, massaging well into patches of psoriasis. Bath next morning to remove excess of product.
- *Side effects:* Sensitivity reactions. The edges of psoriasis patches may become stained purple or brown, but this is not cause for stopping treatment.
- *Special advantages:* Effective non-steroidal treatment of psoriasis.

STEROID PREPARATIONS

Active principal	Proprietary preparation	Formulary preparation
Weak Hydrocortisone	**Alphaderm**	**Hydrocortisone cream** lotion ointment
	Calmurid HC **Cobadex** **Cortacream** **Dioderm** **Dome-Cort** **Efcortelan** **Hydrocortistab** **Hydrocortisyl** **Hydrocortone**	
Hydrocortisone acetate	**Hydrocortistab** **Hydrocortone**	**Hydrocortisone acetate ointment**
Moderately potent Flurandrenolone	**Haelan**	

Clobetasone	Eumovate	Clobetasone cream ointment	
Potent Betamethasone	**Betnovate** **Propaderm**	(various preparations) (various preparations)	
Diflucortolone	**Nerisone** **Temetex**	(various preparations) (various preparations)	
Fluclorolone	**Topilar**	(various preparations)	
Fluocinolone	**Synalar**	(various preparations)	
Fluocinonide	**Metosyn**	(various preparations)	
Fluocortolone	**Ultradil** **Ultralanum**	(various preparations) (various preparations)	
Hydrocortisone butyrate	**Locoid**	(various preparations)	
Triamcinolone acetonide	**Adcortyl** **Ledercort**	(various preparations) (various preparations)	
Very potent Clobetasol	**Dermovate**	(various preparations)	
Halcinonide	**Halciderm** **Halcort**	(various preparations) (various preparations)	

- *Basic precautions:* It is never a good idea to borrow or try somebody else's medicines or preparations. This is particularly true for steroid creams. Steroids used locally are helpful in suppressing the disease process which lies behind troublesome eczemas and psoriasis. But they are in no way curative. Each preparation has to be chosen and prescribed for the individual patient.
- *Proper usage:* Use as little of the preparation as possible to suppress symptoms and use for as short a time as possible. A relatively high relapse rate is noted when use is discontinued.
- *Side effects:* These are roughly equivalent to the strength of the preparation, the amount used and the duration of treatment. The weak and moderately potent preparations rarely cause serious side effects. However, these could be—spread of any local infection; thinning of the skin (which may be permanent); irreversible skin striae (under the skin, not unlike the stretch marks of pregnancy); increased hair growth; blistering around mouth; acne.

Apart from the preparations prescribed, a bewildering number of multiple-mix preparations are available—mostly composed of steroids and antibiotics. It is doubtful whether they are any more effective than the prescriptions described. Readers who wish to assess their relative usefulness or drawbacks can refer to the information on their components as detailed in this chapter. Possibly in no other area of medicine is unjustified polypharmacy so much in evidence.

Chapter

7

TREATING DISORDERS OF SEXUAL FUNCTION

This is one of the areas of modern medicine which has seen a fair amount of growth. Nevertheless, in certain fields (especially impotence) the much sought-after remedy remains elusive, possibly because behavioural, rather than pharmaceutical, factors are so often involved. Because of the effect of medication on hormonal balance—and indeed on the entire system—all treatments are prescription-only and carried on under the supervision of the doctor.

Treatment for sexual dysfunction is considered under five main headings:

Remedies for infertility in the male;
Remedies for infertility in the female;
Remedies for menopausal symptoms;
The treatment of male and female sexual problems;
Hypersexuality therapy.

Remedies for infertility: the male

All remedies discussed in this section are available only on prescription. Many are given in injection form and these are outside the scope of this book.

Hormone treatment of infertility will only be offered after a thorough investigation of the patient's endocrine state. Various forms of treatment can be followed. They include 'rebound' therapy in which large doses of male sex hormones are given to change the internal environment of the testes when function is abnormal. On cessation of treatment, on occasion, a fleeting return to higher sperm counts and greater fertility occurs. This treatment is highly individual and is therefore not covered in this chapter. Another form of treatment is androgen replacement treatment. This may be effective when the patient's testosterone levels are low. In both cases intramuscular injections and tablets by mouth are given. Sometimes pituitary gland problems bring about infertility and recent evidence shows that infection in the urinary tract can be a factor as well.

REPLACEMENT THERAPY

METHYLTESTOSTERONE
Virormone

MESTEROLONE
Pro-Viron
- *Basic precautions:* Caution advised for patients with kidney or liver disease, circulation problems, epilepsy and migraine. Not indicated for use when patient suffers from prostate or breast cancer or nephrosis.
- *Proper dosage:* 10 mg daily for three months (methyltestosterone); 25 mg twice daily (mesterolone).
- *Side effects:* Increase in weight.
- *Special advantages:* Mesterolone is thought to supplement any natural sex hormone and is believed not to affect the liver.

REMEDIES THAT COMBAT INFECTION
It has been shown recently that male infertility is produced by low-grade infection of the urinary tract. In such cases cotrimoxazole, in the forms of Septrin or Bactrim, are used (*see* pages 64–65).

REMEDIES FOR HYPOFERTILITY IN THE MALE
A special type of male infertility is characterised by very low sperm counts. This pregerminal hypofertility may respond to a remedy called clomiphene citrate (Clomid) that was developed as a treatment for certain types of female infertility.

CLOMIPHENE CITRATE
Clomid
- *Basic precautions:* Not suitable for patients with a history or presence of liver disease. Some patients develop blurring of vision or other visual symptoms when taking Clomid, in which case treatment must be abandoned.
- *Proper dosage:* 25 mg daily for one year or until partner conceives.
- *Side effects:* Flushing of face and abdominal discomfort.
- *Special advantages:* Pregnancy rates of 42 per cent have been recorded.

Remedies for infertility: the female

Detailed investigations, usually at a fertility clinic, are mandatory before treatment for infertility in a woman can be prescribed. The approach is to use drugs that act at various levels in the reproductive tract.

THE VAGINA AND CERVIX (NECK OF THE WOMB)
Infection with fungus, yeast, trichomonas or with other more generally infectious germs may reduce fertility. Treatment in such cases is as that for general control of infection. (*See* Chapter 4.)

THE OVARIES

If tests show that the ovaries are not releasing egg cells regularly, or not at all, various solutions may be sought, depending on diagnosis of the essential biological defect. Among preparations known to stimulate the ovaries are:

CLOMIPHENE CITRATE
Clomid

- *Basic precautions:* Not suitable for patients with liver disease, known to have ovarian cysts, or those with abnormal vaginal bleeding or cancer. Not to be used if there is any possibility that the patient is already pregnant.
- *Proper dosage:* 50 mg per day for five days. Repeated at monthly intervals, if necessary, for three months.
- *Side effects:* Blurring of vision (if this occurs treatment should be stopped and patient should see ophthalmologist). Multiple pregnancy (about 7 per cent of Clomid takers), hot flushes, vague abdominal discomfort. Birth defects in children (58 defects reported in 2369 'Clomid' births).
- *Special advantages:* Offers a hope of pregnancy for certain types of ovarian infertility. About 50 per cent of such women become pregnant after 1–3 treatment cycles. Sometimes clomiphene treatment is combined with other therapies (oestrogen or ascorbic acid—vitamin C).

BROMOCRIPTINE
Parlodel

- *Basic precautions:* Prior investigation to exclude pituitary tumour must be carried out prior to therapy. Care if driving or operating machinery, or if a history of severe psychological problems exist.
- *Proper dosage:* Doses of 7.5 mg in divided doses are generally effective, but up to 30 mg per day may be necessary. Usually treatment is started with smaller doses of 1.25 mg at bedtime for three days, then 2.5 mg at bedtime. Dosage is then increased by 1.25 mg taken with meals at two- to three-day intervals until the required dosage is achieved. Often special blood tests indicate required dosage. Treatment is withdrawn after the first missed period.
- *Side effects:* Nausea, dizziness, headache, vomiting, constipation are occasionally reported.
- *Special advantages:* When used to restore fertility it is not associated with any incidence of multiple births, birth defects or pregnancy complications.

Management of the menopause

The necessity of treatment for symptoms of the menopause (change of life) is very variable. In about 15 per cent of women no symptoms (other than a cessation of menstruation) occur. Of the remaining 85 per cent, nine out of ten women experience mild symptoms that do not interfere with their normal lives. Only one woman in ten in this group seeks or needs medical advice. Whether or not treatment of menopausal symptoms ultimately helps the patient is not entirely certain. A minority of medical opinion believes that, although various treatments reduce the intensity of symptoms, the total duration of such symptoms is prolonged. Those doctors who run efficient menopause clinics, however, are more inclined to claim that with suitable treatment the distressing symptoms of the menopause (when these occur) are virtually abolished by treatment. The major areas of symptoms and discomfort are: (1) *local* (vaginal dryness and sexual skin degeneration); (2) *cardiovascular* (heart and blood vessel) changes especially those causing flushing, sweating and palpitation; (3) *psychological* mood changes, depression and anxiety. (These rarely need psychiatric treatment and the various remedies detailed in Chapter 4 may be prescribed.)

LOCAL HORMONE TREATMENTS

● *Basic precautions:* Not to be used during pregnancy or if there is undiagnosed vaginal bleeding, a history of phlebitis, vein thrombosis, or breast tumour. Attempts to discontinue or taper off medication should be made as soon as possible and treatment must not be continued for more than three months without full medical examination.

Preparation	Proper usage
Dienoestrol cream	1–2 applicatorfuls per day for up to two weeks, then reduced gradually
Stilboestrol pessaries	2 pessaries inserted high into vagina at night for two weeks, then reduced
Hormofemin cream	$\frac{1}{2}$–1 applicatorful per day for two weeks, then reduced
Premarin cream	1–2 g per day for three weeks, then at one-week intervals
Tampovagan stilboestrol and Lactic acid	2 pessaries used at night for two weeks, then reduced

HORMONE REPLACEMENT THERAPY (HRT)

When carefully prescribed and properly monitored, many of the remedies are extremely useful in the management of severe menopausal symptoms that do not respond to simpler measures. It must be understood that a similar spectrum of potentially worrying side effects obtain, as are experienced by oral contraceptive users. There are two types of remedy in use: (1) oestrogen (only) remedies, including natural (conjugated) oestrogen; and (2) combined preparations in which oestrogen and progestogen are taken in a sequential manner. More recently the latter preparations have found favour with doctors, mimicking as they do natural hormone surges and recessions. They also seem safer and freer from side effects.

'Simple' oestrogen-only preparations

Active principal	Preparation	Proper dosage
Dienoestrol tablets	**Tablets (F)**	300 micrograms to 5 mg per day for thirty days
Ethinyloestradiol tablets	**Tablets (F)**	10 to 150 micrograms per day for thirty days
Oestradiol	**Progynova**	1–2 mg per day for twenty-one days
Oestriol	**Hormonin Ovestin**	$\frac{1}{2}$–2 tablets per day for twenty days

Conjugated and other oestrogens

Those marketed as 'more natural' oestrogens may have some advantages.

Preparation	Proper dosage
Premarin	Three-strength tablets in twenty-one-day calendar packs are produced. 1 tablet is taken daily for twenty-one days; the cycle is repeated after seven days. The lowest-dose pack necessary to control symptoms is prescribed.
Harmogen	1.5–4.5 mg per day as single dose or divided adjusted to minimum to control symptoms. Maintenance dosage is given for periods of three to four weeks with rest period of five to seven days.
Pentovis	2 capsules twice daily for two to three weeks (only recommended for vaginal discomfort not responding to local treatment—not for routine HRT).

- *Basic precautions:* Not suitable for patients with certain tumours, if there has been a history of vein thrombosis or other clotting disease; in the presence of liver disease, the gynaecological disease endometriosis, or in the rare inherited illness of porphyria.

- *Side effects of 'simple' and 'natural' oestrogen replacement therapy:* Nausea, vomiting, weight gain, breast enlargement and tenderness, 'withdrawal bleeding' (vaginal bleeding after cessation of treatment), fluid retention, jaundice, rashes, depression, headaches. Possibility of causing cancer of womb if treatment is not correctly monitored at clinic.

- *Special advantages:* Usually produces a dramatic improvement of symptoms. Side effects are rare and, provided medical supervision is maintained, risks are few.

Combined preparations (oestrogen plus progestogen)

General note: These preparations, like oral contraceptives, come in calendar packs with strictly defined dosages that, if followed precisely, give very effective responses.

Preparations	Proper dosage
Cyclo-Progynova	1 mg and 2 mg packs
Menophase Prempak Trisequens	0.625 and 1.25 mg packs

- *Basic precautions:* The same general restrictions as apply to the use of oral contraceptives (*see* Chapter 9) should be applied to these remedies. HRT is considered to be a *medical* problem rather than a *social* convenience—contraception could be classed in the latter category—and a greater degree of potential risk is (cheerfully) taken both by the women involved and their doctors. This is somewhat ironic, since the related risks are the same, especially with regards to smoking. Treatment is stopped before surgery or if jaundice occurs. Gynaecological supervision, blood pressure monitoring and regular breast examination are mandatory.

- *Side effects:* Anxiety, increased appetite, fluid retention, breast soreness, palpitating dizziness, depression, dyspepsia, leg pains and migraine (stop treatment), altered sexual appetite, rashes.

- *Special advantages:* These preparations all enjoy the advantages of HRT and, if properly supervised, help many women with severe menopausal problems.

OTHER PREPARATIONS PRESCRIBED FOR MENOPAUSAL SYMPTOMS

Mixogen

This preparation—a blend of oestrogen and testosterone (the male sex hormone androgen) has been used in the management of menopausal symptoms for many decades, often in a remarkably casual way, long before the Pill and classical hormone replacement therapy were introduced. Over the years it has enjoyed a good reputation with reference to side effects, although its potential hazards are similar to all oestrogen/Pill-type remedies. Because it also contains testosterone it does involve potentially worrying virilisation (masculinising) problems.

- *Basic precautions:* As for combined preparations and especially if there is a possibility of pregnancy.
- *Proper dosage:* 1–2 tablets per day for three weeks omitting fourth week; as symptoms settle dosage is reduced.
- *Side effects:* These drugs have side effects similar to those produced by combined pill preparations, but they can also cause hoarseness of voice, acne, growth of facial hair, enlargement of clitoris and elevation of sexual drive (libido). Androgens (which are used in these drugs) are cumulative in their action and virilisation is usually irreversible. Any changes in voice should be an indication to stop treatment.
- *Special advantages:* The continuing popularity (despite its potential hazards) of this preparation indicates its efficacity in menopause management.

CLONIDINE

Dixarit

General note: Unlike previously mentioned compounds to treat the problems of menopause, Dixarit is non-hormonal. It diminishes the liability of the skin vessels to alter their tone and thus prevents the often distressing facial flushing of the menopause. (*See also* use in migraine—Chapter 16.)

- *Basic precautions:* May be unsuitable for some depressed patients. May potentiate antihypertensive therapy.
- *Proper dosage:* 2 tablets twice daily. If no response is obtained in two weeks, increase to 3 tablets twice daily.
- *Side effects:* Sedation, dry mouth, rarely dizziness, disturbed sleep and rashes.
- *Special advantages:* May be used when hormones are to be avoided.

The treatment of sexual problems

The treatment of sexual problems generally falls into two categories. It may be to clear up an infection locally in which case an antifungal or other remedy for vaginal infection may be prescribed (*see* Chapter 4, pages 67–70). Treatment may involve counselling techniques which are, of course, outside the scope of this book. There are, however, a handful of remedies that are regularly prescribed in this context. The treatment of female sexual dysfunction (loss of sexual interest, low libido) sometimes involves taking the male sex hormone testosterone.

TESTOSTERONE
Testoral Sublings
(Tablets to be placed under the tongue.)

- *Basic precautions:* Not suitable for patients with heart disease and breast disease; not to be taken while breast feeding or if suffering from certain kidney diseases, epilepsy, migraine or high blood pressure.
- *Proper dosage:* 1–3 'subling' tablets placed under the tongue and allowed to dissolve.
- *Side effects:* Possibly hoarseness of voice, acne, excessive growth of facial hair, enlargement of clitoris. Any indication of these side effects calls for an immediate cessation of treatment.
- *Special advantages:* In certain intractable cases where other treatments fail this form of hormone treatment is very worthwhile.

Another drug that is being prescribed today in sexual medicine is bromocriptine. Its uses include inhibition of lactation and the treatment of certain cases of erectile failure (impotence) and loss of sexual interest in the female. It is only prescribed when these are shown, by means of a special series of blood tests, to be due to high levels of the hormone prolactin within the body (*see* page 100).

One of the more common of male sexual dysfunctions is premature ejaculation—a condition in which, under the stress of sexual excitement, the man ejaculates his semen before his partner is sufficiently aroused—or even before penetration takes place. Although the consensus of opinion is that counselling is the treatment of choice, a wide variety of drugs have been prescribed. These include reserpine (which is also prescribed to lower the blood pressure, not within the scope of this book), tricyclic antidepressants (*see* Chapter 15, pages 160–164) and Melleril (*see* Chapter 15, page 168).

Remedies used to treat hypersexuality

Occasionally men seek remedies to reduce the level of their sexual drive. This usually happens in cases where previous sexual activity has led to crime and subsequent police action. These remedies are referred to as antiandrogens, being antagonistic to the action of the male sex hormone testosterone.

CYPROTERONE
Androcur
- *Basic precautions:* Not suitable for patients with liver disease.
- *Proper dosage:* 1 tablet twice daily.
- *Side effects:* A decrease in sperm volume, tiredness and lassitude, enlargement of breasts.
- *Special advantages:* An unique remedy for suppression of sexual drive in the male, the effects of which are only experienced when treatment is being taken.

Chapter

8

REMEDIES TO OVERCOME WORM INFESTATIONS

Although this book does not deal in detail with children's remedies, because worm infestations may involve adults too, they are covered below.

Threadworm remedies

Sometimes known as pinworms or seatworms, threadworm infestation is very common—up to 40 per cent of schoolchildren have these worms. Females leave the bowel at the anus at night, lay between 10 to 15,000 eggs, then die. The eggs are very tough and resistant and can survive for several weeks. It is the presence of the female worms while they are laying their eggs that causes itching. The eggs are transferred by the fingers to food and mouth. Infestation is quite common within a family and then becomes a family affair.

Preparations commonly used

PIPERAZINE

▲ Piperazine Elix, Antepar, Pripsen

- *Basic precautions:* If there is a medical history of abnormal kidney function (operations, stones, infection, kidney failure), psychiatric illness, or neurological illness check with doctor. Not suitable for patients with epilepsy and liver disease. Store medicines away from light, below 25°C, in a dry place.
- *Proper usage:* Accurate adherence to dosage is essential. Overdosage will produce side effects, underdosage will not bring about a cure. Hygienic precautions (nail scrubbing after use of lavatory and before meals, and a morning bath) are necessary aids to successful treatment. Piperazine Elix and Antepar tablets and elixir— 1 dose per day for seven days, according to following considerations:

Age	Weight	Elixir		Tablets
Adults	Over 55 kg	15 ml		4
Children				
over thirteen	Over 40 kg	15 ml		4
five to twelve	17–40 kg	10 ml		3
two to four	13–16 kg	5 ml		1½
below two	Below 13 kg		Ask doctor	

Pripsen—a powder packed in sachets which when mixed with water or milk makes a red-coloured drink. 1 dose only with follow-up dose two weeks later. Adults and children over six, 1 sachet; children one to six, $\frac{2}{3}$ sachet; infants three months to one year, $\frac{1}{3}$ sachet.

- *Side effects:* Overdosage may produce dizziness, odd skin sensations (pins and needles), uncoordinated muscular movements, skin rash (urticaria, hives).
- *Special advantages:* As doses are separated by two weeks, side effects are rare. Pripsen contains a senna laxative: the piperazine paralyses the worms which are then evacuated by the senna. Some threadworms may be retained in the bowel in a larval stage. These are removed by the second dose.

MEBENDAZOLE
Vermox
- *Basic precautions:* Is not safe for use by pregnant women. Should not be given to children under the age of two. Suspension should be well shaken before use.
- *Proper usage:* As for piperazine derivatives.
- *Side effects:* Abdominal pain, diarrhoea in rare cases.
- *Special advantages:* Single dose remedy (tablet or suspension) for all ages.

THIABENDAZOLE
Mintezol
Due to multiplicity of side effects this prescription is rarely used for threadworms. It remains a useful 'broad-spectrum' antiworm drug, however (*see* Multiple worm infestation, page 108).

Roundworm remedies

This kind of worm infection vies with threadworm as a common infestation. The roundworm resembles an earthworm—one worm develops from each egg swallowed in 'dirt' or uncooked, soil-contaminated food. The worm lives for about one year in the bowel; the female lays 200,000 eggs per day. Once the eggs are ingested, however, worms do not reproduce inside bowel. They have a complicated life cycle in the host and pass through lungs and circulatory system, eventually becoming mature in bowel.

PIPERAZINE
(*see* threadworms, previous page)
General note: A larger single dose (4 g piperazine hydrate) is recommended and so side effects may be more evident.

BEPHENIUM
▲ Alcopar
- *Basic precautions:* Not recommended for patients who are suffering from vomiting.
- *Proper usage:* The correct dose should be mixed in water or sweet liquid and drunk immediately.
- *Proper dosage:* Adults and children over two years, 1 sachet; children under two years or under 10 kg body weight, $\frac{1}{2}$ sachet.
- *Side effects:* Nausea, vomiting and abdominal discomfort. No serious side effects.

Hookworm remedies

These bloodsucking worms live in the small bowel and if infestation is high, they may cause anaemia. This sometimes has to be treated after worms have been expelled.

Preparations commonly used

TETRACHLOROETHYLENE

▲ Tetrachloroethylene capsules BP

- *Basic precautions:* Not to be used for small or sick children or patients with liver disease. No alcoholic drinks for twenty-four hours before taking medicine.
- *Proper usage:* Take on empty stomach in the morning after eating light meal previous evening.
- *Proper dosage:* Each capsule usually contains 1.0 ml of drug. Take 1–3 capsules as single dose.
- *Side effects:* Giddiness, inebriation and occasionally loss of consciousness. This medicine is similar to chloroform chemically, thus its side effects can be mildly anaesthetic.

▲ Bephenium

(*see* roundworms, opposite)

BITOSCANATE

▲ Bitoscanate BP

- *Basic precautions:* Alcohol and coffee should be avoided at time of treatment.
- *Proper usage:* Treatment should not be repeated until three weeks have elapsed.
- *Proper dosage:* Children five to nine years—2 doses of 50 mg at twelve-hour intervals; children ten to fourteen years—2 doses of 100 mg at twelve-hour intervals; adults—3 doses of 100 mg at twelve-hour intervals.
- *Side effects:* Headaches, giddiness, abdominal pains.

THIABENDAZOLE
(*see* multiple worm infestation, page 108)

Tapeworm remedies

There are several types of tapeworms and diagnosis of the exact worm present is important. This can be done at a hospital laboratory by examining a segment of worm passed in motions. Only after diagnosis should treatment commence as the drug must be matched to the type of tapeworm.

Preparations commonly used

NICLOSAMIDE

▲ Yomesan

- *Basic precautions:* The doctor must be certain that the infestation is not *Taenia solium* (pork tapeworm) as partial digestion of this worm can cause subsequent problems. Laxative should be taken two hours after treatment.

● *Proper usage:* Tablets should be thoroughly chewed before swallowing.

● *Proper dosage:* Children under one year—1 tablet; children two to six years—2 tablets; ages six years to adult—4 tablets.

● *Side effects:* Occasional lightheadedness, bowel overaction, itching around back passage.

MEPACRINE
▲ Mepacrine tablets BP

● *Basic precautions:* The day before dose is to be taken a semi-solid fat-free diet is necessary. The patient must fast overnight. A saline purge (Epsom Salts) is given before taking the tablets. A second saline purge is given one to two hours after last dose.

● *Proper usage:* Adults—4 doses (2 tablets of 100 mg each time) are taken at ten-minute intervals. A drink containing 600 mg of bicarbonate of soda is given to wash down each dose. This minimises side effects. Children to consult doctor for age-related dose.

● *Side effects:* Nausea and vomiting if the bicarbonate is omitted.

Multiple worm infestation remedies (threadworms, roundworms, hookworms)

In some parts of the world (eg the subcontinent of India and Africa) multiple worm infestation is common. Visitors or immigrants may suffer in this way. One drug is commonly used:

THIABENDAZOLE
▲ Mintezol

● *Basic precautions:* Not suitable for patients with kidney or liver disease, or for those who drive or operate machinery.

● *Proper usage:* Tablets should be taken with meals.

● *Proper dosage:*

Weight	kg	lb	Dose twice daily
	10	22	$\frac{1}{2}$ tablet
	20	44	1 tablet
	30	66	$1\frac{1}{2}$ tablets
	40	88	2 tablets
	50	110	$2\frac{1}{2}$ tablets
	60+	132+	3 tablets

● *Side effects:* Loss of appetite, nausea, vomiting and dizziness. More rarely stomach pain, diarrhoea, headache, drowsiness, irritation around back passage. Some patients notice a strange smell to their urine after therapy.

9

CONTRACEPTION

Contraception, in the modern sense, has a short history and only quite recently has reached a high degree of efficiency. Broadly speaking, the subject divides itself into contraceptive practices for the male (an efficient enough method that remains outside the provisions of the Health Service) and methods that involve the female partner. There are, of course, measures that come outside the scope of this book (sterilisation, injectable and 'natural' contraceptive practices).

Contraception for the male—the condom

Modern condoms (sheaths/French letters) are made of a thin stretchable latex film. Reputable brands like Durex products are manufactured under careful conditions of quality control, and when properly stored have a long 'shelf-life'. 'Fancy' products sold extensively in sex shops and through certain mail order companies may be unreliable. Male contraceptive products are not available on the National Health Service.

- *Basic precautions:* The only known contraindication to condom usage is the very rare sensitivity reaction to the latex used in manufacture.
- *Proper usage:* The condom must be applied to the erect penis before vaginal penetration takes place and removed from the penis before the erection subsides. In the case of sexual neophytes some suitable lubricant should be applied to the unsheathed penis or to the female sexual parts before penetration is attempted.
- *Special advantages:* Easy (non-medical) availability, freedom from side effects, protection against most venereal disease (including herpes). It is possible it provides some protection against the formation of cervical carcinoma in women.
- *Efficiency:* Contraceptive failure rates are based on the number of pregnancies occurring in one year when one hundred women use the contraceptive in question. Patient motivation and care of usage are important factors in failure rates. This is particularly the case in condom usage. A failure rate as high as five (pregnancies per one hundred woman-years) has been reported; in other studies failure rates as low as 0.4 have been demonstrated. Very few condom failures are due to mechanical reasons (damaged or imperfect condoms). It is almost invariably improper usage that is responsible for failure in this case.

Contraception for the female

SPERMICIDES

Until newer methods of female contraception evolved, spermicides were an important method of contraception. Now they are largely used as back-up contraceptives either in conjunction with condom usage or with barrier methods of female contraception. Originally, a wide variety of spermicidal chemicals were used. Now only two efficient spermicides—nonoxynol and di-isobutylphenoxypolyethoxyethanol ('di-iso') are present in modern ethical products.

NONOXYNOL PRODUCTS

▲ **C-Film**

A unique product in that it is a 5 cm square film to be inserted into vagina fifteen minutes to one hour before intercourse. It is said to be effective within one minute.

▲ **Delfen**—Cream or foam aerosol

▲ **Duracreme**—Cream

▲ **Duragel**—Gel

▲ **Emko**—Aerosol foam

▲ **Genexol**—Pessary (not to be used with vaginal barrier contraception)

▲ **Ortho-Creme**—Cream

▲ **Ortho-Forms**—Pessary

▲ **Rendells**—Pessary (not to be used with vaginal barrier contraception)

▲ **Staycept**—Pessary or jelly

DI-ISO PRODUCT

▲ **Ortho-Gynol jelly**

- *Basic precautions:* Sensitivity in rare cases prohibits use.
- *Proper usage:* The type of spermicide used in many cases determines proper usage. Pessaries—should be inserted high into the vagina at least fifteen minutes before intercourse takes place. Creams—these tend to remain where they are put in the vagina rather than spreading as do pessaries, jellies, gels and foam tablets. Especial care of insertion (through an applicator) is mandatory for most efficient usage. Gels, jellies and pastes, foam tablets—rapid action in the protection afforded. Foam aerosols—need to be injected high into vagina.
- *Side effects:* Jellies and pastes have a high 'leakage' factor and foams may appear in quantity at entrance to vagina. No long-term side effects known.
- *Special advantages:* Free availability. Disadvantages—poor efficiency (nine to sixty-two failures per one hundred woman-user years). Some women have difficulty using them properly even when excellent manufacturers' leaflets are available.

BARRIER DEVICES

These have to be fitted by doctors *au fait* with modern contraceptive practice. Various types of devices are in use:

▲ The Dumas vault device, the vaginal diaphragm, the vimule and the cervical cap

The fitting physician ascertains which is the most suitable and prescribes accordingly.

- *Basic precautions:* Devices that prove effective at one time in a woman's life may not be reliable at a later stage (after a pregnancy). Similarly, a gynaecological problem may supervene and alter her internal anatomy.
- *Proper usage:* The device and appropriate spermicide should be inserted before coitus commences. If coitus is repeated after six hours then spermicide needs to be reapplied if high efficiency is to be retained. In some women bowel movement may alter the position of the diaphragm. All women using barrier devices are taught how to fit the device themselves and to check that the device is in the proper position in the vagina.
- *Side effects:* None, other than personal psychological or aesthetic objections.
- *Proper storage:* Modern barrier devices have a long life provided they are washed, rinsed and dried after use, kept in a cool place and not used in conjunction with spermicides that are unsuitable.
- *Special advantages:* Freedom from side effects. Failure rates of about 2.4 per one hundred woman-user years are reported but with high motivation this may well be halved.

HORMONAL CONTRACEPTION

The Pill, in its various forms, has transformed contraceptive practice and several types of Pill are in common use, although all prescription-only. Many women taking the Pill have only the haziest knowledge of the type of Pill they are using. It will be one of the following types.

Combined Pill: It is called 'combined' because each Pill contains both an oestrogen and a progestogen. This may be in fixed dosage (as in most Pills) or in 'phasic' form in which the relative amounts of oestrogen and progestogen vary throughout the month. Within the combined Pill range, groups of Pills are often designated by the amount of oestrogen each Pill contains and so 20, 30, 35 and 50 microgram Pills are prescribable. It is *usually* easy for the taker to know if they are on a combined Pill because usually there is a six- or seven-day interval during administration when no Pills are taken. The word 'usually' is in italics because sometimes in an attempt to rule out confusion over Pill-less days (a factor that confuses or worries some women), some manufacturers produce 'everyday' (ED) packs of combined Pills in which seven of the twenty-eight pills are hormoneless (dummy) tablets.

Progestogen-only contraceptives: These Pills only contain one hormone, a progestogen. They can be usually (*see* above) distinguished from combined Pills by the fact that no Pill-less days exist and the regime of Pill-taking once started has to be maintained continually while contraceptive cover is required.

The combined-Pill oral contraception
Although the prescribing physician is responsible for excluding all medical contra-indications to Pill prescription, this matter is so important that it is detailed here in the same detail as any other prescription-only item is dealt with in this book.

The fact that there are nearly thirty combined Pills on the market is evidence of the fact that some Pills are better for some people than others. The factors that influence doctors' prescriptions are legion. But the following factors are generally carefully evaluated.

Oestrogen content: This varies from 20 (extra low) to 50 micrograms (medium) per Pill (high dose Pills of over 50 micrograms of oestrogen per Pill have now been withdrawn). Doctors, generally speaking, tend to prescribe the least possible dose of oestrogen compatible with contraceptive efficiency and good cycle control. The latter phrase means that vaginal bleeding occurs regularly on day twenty-two and lasts for a few days. Spotting or more vigorous breakthrough bleeding, mid-cycle, is evidence of poor control and probably, incidentally, less than efficient contraception. Sometimes unless Pill taking is precisely timed—say at 11 pm, and not between 10 and 12 pm each night, cycle control is poor. Again this probably means that the oestrogen content of the Pill is less than adequately prescribed and a higher oestrogen Pill is then prescribed.

Progestogen content: Until comparatively recently the amount of progestogen, and the type of progestogen in contraceptive Pills, was not thought to be of much importance. Now there is a much greater emphasis being placed on progestogen dose and chemistry. There is a fairly large range of progestogens that have a contraceptive action.

Phasic formulation: The introduction, initially, of the triphasic oral contraceptives and later biphasic ones has come about as an attempt to produce Pills that more closely reflect the normal physiology of the female reproductive tract. Unlike the other combined Pills they are started on day one of the cycle (onset of period).

Everyday (ED) dosage: To offset women being confused or forgetful about combined Pill taking, this pack allows for a Pill-a-day regime to be followed. Some doctors feel they can identify the woman who needs such a pack.

Combined Pill contraceptives include:

Anovlar 21, norethisterone acetate 4 mg, ethinyloestradiol 50 micrograms

Bi Novum (calendar pack), 7 white tablets norethisterone 0.5 mg plus 35 micrograms ethinyloestradiol and 14 peach tablets 1.0 mg norethisterone plus 35 micrograms ethinyloestradiol

Brevinor, norethisterone 500 micrograms, ethinyloestradiol 35 micrograms

Conova 30, ethynodiol diacetate 2 mg, ethinyloestradiol 30 micrograms

Eugynon 30, levonorgestrel 250 micrograms, ethinyloestradiol 30 micrograms

Eugynon 50, norgestrel 500 micrograms, ethinyloestradiol 50 micrograms

Gynovlar 21, norethisterone acetate 3 mg, ethinyloestradiol 50 micrograms

Loestrin 20, norethisterone acetate 1 mg, ethinyloestradiol 20 micrograms

Logynon (calendar pack): 6 tablets levonorgestrel 50 micrograms, ethinyloestradiol 30 micrograms; 5 tablets levonorgestrel 75 micrograms, ethinyloestradiol 40 micrograms; 10 tablets levonorgestrel 125 micrograms, ethinyloestradiol 30 micrograms
Dosage: 1 tablet per day for twenty-one days, starting with tablet marked 1 on first day of cycle, and repeated after a seven-day interval

Logynon ED, as for Logynon; in addition 7 placebo tablets

Marvelon, desogestrel 0.150 mg, ethinyloestradiol 0.03 mg

Microgynon 30, levonorgestrel 150 micrograms, ethinyloestradiol 30 micrograms

Minilyn, lynoestrenol 2.5 mg, ethinyloestradiol 50 micrograms
Dosage: 1 tablet per day for twenty-two days, starting on fifth day of cycle, and repeated after a six-day interval

Minovlar, norethisterone acetate 1 mg, ethinyloestradiol 50 micrograms

Minovlar ED, as for Minovlar; in addition 7 placebo tablets

Norimin, norethisterone 1 mg, ethinyloestradiol 35 micrograms

Norinyl-1, norethisterone 1 mg, nestranol 50 micrograms

Norlestrin, norethisterone acetate 2.5 mg, ethinyloestradiol 50 micrograms

Orlest 21, norethisterone acetate 1 mg, ethinyloestradiol 50 micrograms

Ortho-Novin 1/50, norethisterone 1 mg, mestranol 50 micrograms

Ovran, levonorgestrel 250 micrograms, ethinyloestradiol 50 micrograms

Ovran 30, levonorgestrel 250 micrograms, ethinyloestradiol 30 micrograms

Ovranette, levonorgestrel 150 micrograms, ethinyloestradiol 30 micrograms

Ovulen 50, ethynodiol diacetate 1 mg, ethinyloestradiol 50 micrograms

Ovysmen, norethisterone 500 micrograms, ethinyloestradiol 35 micrograms

Trinordiol (calendar pack): 6 tablets levonorgestrel 50 micrograms, ethinyloestradiol 30 micrograms; 5 tablets levonorgestrel 75 micrograms, ethinyloestradiol 40 micrograms; 10 tablets levonorgestrel 125 micrograms, ethinyloestradiol 30 micrograms
Dosage: 1 tablet per day for twenty-one days, starting with tablet marked 1 on first day of cycle, and repeated after a seven-day interval.

- *Basic precautions:* Not suitable if the possibility of pregnancy exists, or if patient has, or has previously suffered from, vein or other blood vessel thrombosis, acute or chronic liver disease, jaundice or severe pruritus (itching), known or suspected breast cancer, or hormone-dependent cancer, or undiagnosed vaginal bleeding. High blood pressure and obesity may well exclude taking as well. Not suitable for lactating women.

● *Proper supervision:* High blood pressure (usually reversible after discontinuance) occurs rarely in Pill takers and so routine monitoring of blood pressure is mandatory. An increased risk of coronary disease occurs in Pill takers on rare occasions. It is exacerbated by other predisposing factors including cigarette smoking, obesity, diabetes, a history of several pregnancies, toxaemia and age (over thirty-five). Patients suffering from epilepsy, migraine, asthma or heart disease may find symptoms are exacerbated by Pill taking. Diabetics may need special control. Pill takers should undergo regular pelvic and breast examination.

Gastrointestinal upsets, and some drugs, may modify effectiveness of Pill (especially sedatives, antibiotics, antiepileptic and antiarthritic drugs).

Special supervision is advised if the taker has suffered from breast lumps, depression, varicose veins, anaemia, diabetes, blood pressure, epilepsy, asthma, otosclerosis, multiple sclerosis, porphyria, gall stones, chloasma and herpes. Contact lenses may become uncomfortable. (Through a lapse in precautions, a Pill taker may find herself pregnant. She should, of course, report to her doctor and inform him of her Pill-taking history.)

Pills should be discontinued at least six weeks prior to surgery or if immobilisation (eg plaster cast) is necessary.

Women who have irregular menstrual cycles may bleed regularly while on Pill but revert to their previous state, or may more permanently lose their periods after Pill taking. This may be associated with subsequent reduced fertility or infertility. All women over thirty-five need special supervision if they are Pill takers.

● *Proper dosage:* The first day of the menstrual flow is taken as day one when referring to Pill-taking regimes. In most packs 21 Pills form one pack. The first Pill is taken on day five and repeated until the daily pack is empty. Then no Pills are taken for seven days. (ED—in everyday packs dummy tablets are taken during the seven days.) A new pack is recommended twenty-nine days after day one and this sequence is maintained indefinitely while contraceptive cover is required.

During the first cycle (first pack) of Pill taking, an additional method of contraception is necessary for the first fourteen days of Pill taking. On the second (and subsequent packs) this is not necessary.

● *Forgotten tablets:* To get the most efficient results, regular daily dosage is mandatory and for 'low-dosage' Pills (*see* page 112) this should also be hour-specific (ie at the same time of day). If a tablet is missed it should be taken as soon as possible. If 2 tablets are missed, an extra tablet should be taken and an additional contraceptive method practised for the rest of the cycle. If more than 2 tablets are missed the Pill should be abandoned and other contraceptive cover be used. The next cycle of Pill taking should be treated as a first cycle (*see* above).

● *Pill changing:* Any new combined Pill should be started seven days after finishing a pack of a previous combined Pill. This should be treated once again as a first cycle.

● *After childbirth, miscarriage or abortion:* The combined Pill is not suitable for lactating women. Unless Pill taking starts, with medical sanction seven days after delivery, Pill taking commences once menstruation is resumed. Other contraceptive cover in the meanwhile is necessary if an unwanted pregnancy is to be avoided in these cases.

● *Side effects:* Slight transient nausea, weight gain, breast discomfort usually disappear after first cycle. Loss of libido occurs occasionally. Spotting or bleeding may occur at any time during the first few cycles. This may indicate too low a dosage and a change of Pill could be indicated. Such symptoms, however, may be due to irregular Pill taking. Occasionally no bleeding occurs during Pill-free or dummy-tablet days. Medical information should be sought if this occurs but it is rarely a sign of pregnancy.

● *Special advantages:* The combined Pill, when efficiently taken, is associated with a negligible failure rate and it is for most women an ideal contraceptive.

Progestogen-only contraception

As previously mentioned, such Pills contain no oestrogen. The progestogen used varies and several different progestogens are currently used. These are argued to have rather different side effects and safety factors, but to a large extent these are in dispute at the time of writing, and the following is a broad outline of their use.

Progestogen-only Pills include:

Femulen, ethynodiol diacetate 500 micrograms

Micronor, norethisterone 350 micrograms

Microval, levonorgestrel 30 micrograms

Neogest, norgestrel 75 micrograms

Norgeston, levonorgestrel 30 micrograms

Noriday, norethisterone 350 micrograms

● *Basic precautions:* Not suitable for women with liver disease or who have been jaundiced, unless liver function tests are normal. Not suitable for those who have undiagnosed vaginal bleeding or if possibility of pregnancy exists. Not suitable in the presence of certain blood-clotting disorders (thrombo-embolism). Special care in migraine if being treated with vaso-constricting drug (*see* pages 185–188), especially Dixarit, Deseril, Midrid and the ergotamines.

● *Proper management:* This follows a similar pattern to that detailed on page 112 for combined-Pill management. The following side effects dictate immediate discontinuance of Pill:

(i) loss of vision, double vision or any worrying visual symptom;

(ii) worsening of migraine or severe headache;

(iii) any serious unexplained illness.

● *Proper dosage:* Tablets start on the first day of menstruation and are continued without interruption while contraceptive effect is required. They should be taken at the same time of day and preferably in the evening. If a time space between Pill taking exceeds twenty-seven hours their efficiency is reduced. During the first fourteen days of Pill taking alternative back-up contraception is advised. If Pills are missed no extra Pills should be taken, but back-up contraception should be used for 14 days.

If a woman should vomit after Pill taking, another Pill should be taken within three hours to maintain contraception. If repeated gastroenteritis ensues, back-up contraception is necessary for fourteen days after symptoms settle.

Should a change be made from the combined Pill to a progestogen-only Pill, women should have seven Pill-free days after taking the last combined Pill, and then start the progestogen-only Pill. Back-up contraception should continue for fourteen days. Antibiotics, antiepileptic drugs and sedatives may reduce efficiency of Pill.

• *Side effects:* Slight headache, weight gain, nausea, breast tenderness and spotting between periods may occur, but diminish with use. Previous menstrual patterns and regular cycles of bleeding may not occur for three or four months after cessation of Pill use. If regular periods do not eventually return medical advice is necessary and may or may not indicate a need for change of contraceptive technique.

• *Special advantages:* Contains no oestrogen, so free from oestrogen-type side effects. This does not mean that no vascular side effects occur. Suitable during breast feeding, suitable for the older woman. Contraceptive efficiency is lower than combined Pill but still high.

Chapter

10

MANAGING ANAEMIA

Anaemia can have many forms but by far the commonest is that caused by iron deficiency. In such cases the body finds itself short of iron and the symptoms of anaemia develop. In the past, iron was popular as a tonic—especially for supposedly 'anaemic' children. Today doctors believe that a diagnosis of anaemia must rest on the result of a blood test—except in certain cases when anaemia tends to occur so frequently that prophylactic (preventative) iron treatment is indicated. This relatively small group of patients includes pregnant women, patients who have had an operation on the stomach (gastrectomy) and low birthweight, premature or Caesarean birth babies. Iron treatment by injection is called for in some exceedingly rare cases.

A condition much rarer than the simple iron deficiency anaemia is megaloblastic anaemia. It is due to a lack of either vitamin B12 or folic acid in the body. If vitamin B12 is the essential problem replacement is necessary by injection; this is outside the scope of this book. If the body is becoming anaemic due to a lack of folic acid this can be given in tablet form. Sometimes both iron and folic acid are deficient and are prescribed together.

Very rare indeed are the hypoplastic and haemolytic anaemias in which medication is a complicated affair and specialised management is always necessary and very variable.

The rationale of iron replacement therapy

Iron is available in many forms for the doctor to prescribe. The aim of efficient treatment is, first of all, to give the body enough iron to build up an optimal level in the blood, and then to replenish its (usually) depleted iron stores. To ensure that the latter objective has been achieved it is necessary to continue with iron medication for six months after a blood count has pronounced that the circulatory blood contains sufficient iron.

Iron, however, can create some side effects. These are universal and include gastrointestinal upset and constipation. The plethora of iron compounds available is evidence of the attempt to produce a tablet with enough elemental iron in it to rapidly cure the anaemia without causing unwanted symptoms. Sometimes a preparation keeps side effects to an acceptable level; many will, however, say that it does so because it sacrifices the quantity of elemental iron it contains per tablet.

In the quest for more efficient iron therapy two reasonably successful devices have been developed. Perhaps the most helpful is the combination of vitamin C and iron in one pill. This seems to increase appreciably the amount of iron absorbed by the body. Less well proven is the slow-release iron tablet which, theoretically, only releases its load of iron once the pill has passed through the stomach, thus preventing gastric irritation by the astringent iron. Critics claim that these preparations often pass through that part of the intestine in which iron is absorbed before the full load of iron can be assimilated, and this reduces their efficiency.

Some iron tablets contain very complex formulations of iron, vitamins, trace elements, liver and various so-called 'tonic' preparations. Scientific fact does not support the rationale for their composition, but in practice many patients find them effective. All preparations are prescription and OTC except those containing folic acid which are available on prescription only.

COMPARATIVE TABLES OF COMPOSITION

General note: To treat an anaemic person 100–200 mg of elemental iron is needed per day. Once anaemia is under control, maintenance therapy may be reduced. Iron-containing compounds used in medicine include various iron salts.

Ferrous fumarate remedies

Preparation (Proprietary or formulary)	Amount of elemental iron
▲ Ferrous fumarate tablet	65 mg
▲ Fersaday tablet	100 mg
▲ Fersamal tablet	65 mg
▲ 5 cc Fersamal syrup	45 mg
▲ Galfer capsule	100 mg

Ferrous gluconate remedies

Preparation	Amount of elemental iron
▲ Ferrous gluconate tablet (300 mg)	36 mg
▲ Fergon tablet (300 mg)	36 mg

Ferrous glycine remedies

Preparation	Amount of elemental iron
▲ Fe-Cap capsule (565 mg)	100 mg
▲ Ferrocontin Continus tablet	100 mg
▲ Kelferon tablet	40 mg
▲ 5 ml Plesmet syrup	25 mg

Ferrous succinate remedies

Preparation	Amount of elemental iron
▲ Ferrous succinate tablet (100 mg)	100 mg
▲ Ferromyn tablet (100 mg)	35 mg
▲ 5 ml Ferromyn elixir	37 mg

Ferrous sulphate remedies

Preparation	Amount of elemental iron
▲ Ferrous sulphate tablet (200 mg)	60 mg
▲ Feospan capsule (150 mg)	45 mg
▲ Ferro-Gradumet tablet (325 mg)	105 mg
▲ 5 ml Ferrous sulphate mixture	12 mg
▲ Slow-Fe tablet (160 mg)	48 mg

Polysaccharide-iron complex tablets

Preparation	Amount of elemental iron
▲ Niferex tablet	50 mg
▲ 5 ml Niferex elixir	100 mg

Sodium iron vedetate

Preparation	Amount of elemental iron
▲ 5 ml Sytron	27.5 mg

- *Principles of treatment:* In general, a total of 100–200 mg of elemental iron are prescribed, to be taken daily (after food) made up of 1 or several dosages. But this may be reduced if intolerance, in the form of gastrointestinal symptoms, occurs. Another preparation may then be tried.

Treatment for anaemia caused by iron and folic acid deficiency in pregnancy

Drugs commonly used

Proprietary preparation	Composition
Co-Ferol Tablets	Ferrous fumarate 120 mg, equivalent to 40 mg ferrous iron, folic acid 200 micrograms
Fe-Cap Folic Capsules	Ferrous glycine sulphate 450 mg, folic acid 350 micrograms
Fefol Spansules	Dried ferrous sulphate 150 mg, folic acid 500 micrograms
Feravol-F Tablets	Ferrous gluconate 300 mg, folic acid 3 mg
Ferrocap-F 350 Capsules	Ferrous fumarate 330 mg, folic acid 350 micrograms

Ferrocontin F Continus Tablets	Ferrous glycine sulphate 562.5 mg, folic acid 500 micrograms
Folex-350 Tablets	Ferrous fumarate 308 mg, folic acid 350 micrograms
Folvron Tablets	Dried ferrous sulphate 194 mg, folic acid 1.7 mg
Galfer FA Capsules	Ferrous fumarate, equivalent to 100 mg ferrous iron, folic acid 350 micrograms
Kelfolate Tablets	Ferrous glycine sulphate 225 mg, folic acid 150 micrograms
Pregaday Tablets	Ferrous fumarate, equivalent to 100 mg ferrous iron, folic acid 350 micrograms
Pregfol Capsules	Ferrous sulphate 270 mg, folic acid 500 micrograms
Slow-Fe Folic Tablets	Dried ferrous sulphate 160 mg, folic acid 400 micrograms

Compound iron preparations

These have a part to play in therapy, particularly if they contain vitamin C which helps iron absorption, or if the doctor is convinced that other vitamin deficiencies are present. Some contain odd additives that are less supportable scientifically.

Drugs commonly used

Proprietary preparation	Composition
▲ Ferrous Sulphate Tablets Compound	Dried ferrous sulphate, an amount equivalent to 170 mg of ferrous sulphate, copper sulphate 2.5 mg, manganese sulphate 2.5 mg
▲ Anorvit Tablets	Acetomenaphthone, ascorbic acid, dried ferrous sulphate
▲ BC 500 with Iron Tablets	Calcium pantothenate, ferrous fumarate, nicotinamide, pyridoxine hydrochloride, riboflavine, sodium ascorbate, thiamine mononitrate
▲ FEAC Tablets	Ascorbic acid, dried ferrous sulphate, nicotinamide, pyridoxine hydrochloride, riboflavine, thiamine mononitrate
▲ Fe-Cap C Capsules	Ascorbic acid, ferrous glycine sulphate
Fefol-Vit Spansules	Ascorbic acid, calcium pantothenate, dried ferrous sulphate, folic acid, nicotinamide, pyridoxine hydrochloride, riboflavine, thiamine mononitrate
▲ Feravol Tablets	Ascorbic acid, dried ferrous sulphate, riboflavine, thiamine hydrochloride
▲ Feravol Syrup	Ascorbic acid, ferrous sulphate, riboflavine, thiamine hydrochloride
▲ Feravol-G Tablets	Ferrous gluconate, thiamine hydrochloride
▲ Feravol-G Syrup	Same ingredients as the tablets
Ferfolic Tablets	Ascorbic acid, ferrous gluconate, folic acid, nicotinamide, riboflavine, thiamine hydrochloride
Ferfolic SV Tablets	Ascorbic acid, ferrous gluconate, folic acid

▲ Fergluvite Tablets	Ascorbic acid, ferrous gluconate, nicotinamide, riboflavine, thiamine hydrochloride
▲ Ferraplex B Tablets	Ascorbic acid, dried brewer's yeast, copper carbonate, dried ferrous sulphate, nicotinamide, riboflavine, thiamine hydrochloride
▲ Ferrlecit 100 Tablets	Ascorbic acid, dried ferrous sulphate, sodium ferric citrate
▲ Ferrocap Capsules	Ferrous fumarate, thiamine hydrochloride
▲ Ferrograd C Tablets	Dried ferrous sulphate, sodium ascorbate
▲ Ferromyn B Tablets	Ferrous succinate, nicotinamide, riboflavine, thiamine hydrochloride
▲ Ferromyn B Elixir	5 ml elixir = 1 tablet
▲ Ferromyn S Tablets	Ferrous succinate, succinic acid
Ferromyn S Folic Tablets	Ingredients as for Ferromyn S Tablets with addition of folic acid
▲ Fesovit Spansules	Ascorbic acid, calcium pantothenate, dried ferrous sulphate, nicotinamide, riboflavine, pyridoxine hydrochloride, thiamine mononitrate
Folicin Tablets	Copper sulphate, dried ferrous sulphate, folic acid, manganese sulphate
▲ Forceval Capsules	Ascorbic acid, calcium as calcium hydrogen phosphate, calcium pantothenate, chlorine bitartrate, copper, cyanocobalamin, inositol, iodine, iron lysine hydrochloride, magnesium, manganese, nicotinamide, phosphorus, potassium pyridoxine hydrochloride, riboflavine, thiamine mononitrate, vitamin A, vitamin D, vitamin E
▲ Gastrovite Tablets	Ascorbic acid, calciferol, calcium gluconate, ferrous glycine sulphate
▲ Gevral Capsules	Ascorbic acid, calciferol, calcium pantothenate, chlorine bitartrate, copper oxide, cyanocobalamin, ferrous fumarate, inositol, magnesium oxide, manganese dioxide, nicotinamide, potassium iodide, potassium sulphate, pyridoxine hydrochloride, riboflavine, thiamine mononitrate, d-a-topopheryl acetate, vitamin A yeast, zinc oxide
▲ Glykola Elixir	Caffeine, calcium glycerophosphate, ferric chloride solution, kola liquid extract
▲ Iberet 500 Tablets	Ascorbic acid, calcium pantothenate, dried ferrous sulphate, nicotinamide, pyridoxine hydrochloride, riboflavine, thiamine mononitrate
▲ Iberol Filmtabs	Dried ferrous sulphate, liver fraction, nicotinamide, pyridoxine hydrochloride, riboflavine, sodium ascorbate, thiamine mononitrate
Irofol Filmtabs	Dried ferrous sulphate, folic acid, sodium ascorbate
▲ Iron Jelloids	Ferrous sulphate with vitamins B_1, B_2, nicotinamide and C
Ironorm Capsules	Ascorbic acid, cyanocobalamin, dried ferrous sulphate, folic acid, concentrated intrinsic factor, liver fraction, nicotinamide, riboflavine, thiamine hydrochloride

Proprietary preparation	Composition
Ironorm Tonic with Iron	Calcium pantothenate, cyanocobalamin, ferric ammonium citrate, glycerophosphates of calcium manganese, sodium and potassium, nicotinamide, proteolysed liver extract, pyridoxine hydrochloride, thiamine hydrochloride
▲ **Iron Plan**	150 mg ferrous sulphate and 3 mg vitamin B_1
▲ **Minadex Syrup**	Calcium glycerophosphate, copper sulphate, ferric ammonium citrate, manganese sulphate, potassium glycerophosphate, vitamin A, D
▲ **Phillips Iron Tonic**	Ferrous carbonate, yeast, vitamins B_1, B_2 and C
▲ **Phyllosan**	Ferrous fumarate plus nicotinic acid, vitamins B_1, B_2 and C
Pregavite Forte F Tablets	Ascorbic acid, calcium phosphate, dried ferrous sulphate, nicotinamide, pyridoxine hydrochloride, riboflavine, thiamine hydrochloride, vitamin A, D and folic acid
▲ **Sidros Tablets**	Ascorbic acid, ferrous gluconate
▲ **Tonivitan A and D Syrup**	Orange, calciferol, calcium glycerophosphate, copper sulphate, ferrous ammonium citrate, manganese glycerophosphate, vitamin A

Chapter

11

REMEDIES FOR RHEUMATISM

Most so-called rheumatic aches and pains are unrelated to any of the established rheumatic diseases. These symptoms, which tend to be referred to as fibrositis, 'the screws', myalgia or muscular rheumatism, are, nevertheless, quite painful and worthy of treatment. Some of the real rheumatic diseases are acute and dramatic— for instance gout. Such diseases are, generally speaking, the most easily curable.

Managing 'rheumatic' arthritis

Many rheumatic diseases are chronic and arthritic in nature. They are associated with general ill health and mounting disability. In some cases they are a life-long problem and they rarely respond to one particular remedy. Since this will be a question of long-term treatment, a truly close yet flexible contact should be maintained between doctor and patient. A real understanding of the chronic nature of rheumatism by both patient and doctor very often establishes a just perspective of the management of the disease. Safe and simple drugs can be thought more appropriate than new and complicated remedies that may still be experimental, or not tested over many years. This is not to say that the most powerful modern drugs are not called for from time to time. One such drug, gold injection therapy, is not dealt with in this chapter because injection treatment allows for no personal modification by the patient. (In other words, the doctor who is giving the injection to the patient is totally responsible for the therapy.)

TREATING RHEUMATIC PAIN

In the fibrositic types of rheumatism self-medication, using simple remedies for pain (*see* Chapter 16), can be quite effective. These can be used with 'rubs' and embrocations.

Liquid rubs

Formulary preparations	Principal ingredients
▲ Methyl Salicylate Liniment	Salicylates

Table continued on next page

Liquid rubs *continued*

Preparations	Principal ingredients
▲ Turpentine Liniment (F)	Camphor, turpentine
▲ White Liniment (F)	Ammonia, turpentine
▲ Aspellin	Camphor, menthol, salicylate
▲ Ellimans Embrocation	Turpentine
▲ Deep Heat Lotion	Menthol, methyl salicylate
▲ Radian B Spirit Liniment	Menthol, salicylate, turpentine, camphor
▲ Sloan's Liniment	Pine oil, salicylate, turpentine, camphor, capsicum

Solid rub

Proprietary preparation	Principal ingredients
▲ Ralgex Stick	Salicylates, capsicum, menthol

Creams and ointments

Formulary preparation	Principal ingredients
▲ Methyl Salicylate Ointment	Salicylates

Proprietary preparations	Principal ingredients
▲ Algesal	Salicylate
▲ Algipan	Capsicum, salicylate, histamine
▲ Aradolene	Salicylate, capsicum, menthol, camphor
▲ Balmosa	Camphor, capsicum, menthol, salicylate, iodine
▲ Bayolin	Nicotinate, salicylate
▲ Bengue's Balsam and SG	Menthol, salicylate
▲ Cremalgex	Capsicum, salicylate, histamine, nicotinate
▲ Cremalgin	Capsicum, salicylate, histamine
▲ Cremathurm	Capsicum, nicotinate, histamine, salicylate
▲ Deep Heat Rub	Menthol, eucalyptus, methyl salicylate, turpentine
▲ Difflam	Benzydamine
▲ Intralgin	Salicylamide, benzocaine
▲ Lloyd's Cream	Salicylates
Movelat	Steroid, salicylate

▲ Radian Massage Cream	Menthol, camphor, salicylates, capsicum
▲ Ralgex Balm	Methyl nicotinate, histamine, capsicum
▲ Transvasin	Benzocaine, nicotinate, salicylate

Aerosols

Proprietary preparations	Principal ingredients
▲ Algispray	Salicylates, methyl nicotinate
▲ Aspellin	Camphor, menthol
▲ Deep Heat	Salicylates, methyl nicotinate
▲ Dubam	Salicylates, nicotinate
▲ PR Spray	Fluoromethanes
▲ Radian B	Salicylates, menthol, camphor
▲ Ralgex	Salicylates, methyl nicotinate
▲ Skefron	Fluoromethanes

- *Basic precautions:* Not to be used if patient is known to be sensitive to any of the ingredients. Not to be applied near mucous surfaces (eye, mouth, vagina, rectum). Not to be used if skin is broken.
- *Proper usage:* Massage in two to three times daily. Aerosols—hold container upright one to two feet from affected area and press button so that jet, not fine spray, is produced. Apply jet to painful area for three to five seconds, repeat after half a minute and once more in another half-minute if necessary. Maximum 3 treatments in one day. Carefully screen eyes, nostrils and mouth.
- *Side effects:* Sensitivity to ingredients occurs infrequently. If rash develops stop treatment. Avoid sunshine after use.
- *Special advantages:* Very helpful, simple pain-relieving treatments that have stood the test of time. They should not be discontinued because their mode of action is not very well understood.

PAINKILLERS THAT ALSO REDUCE RHEUMATIC INFLAMMATION

Aspirin and salicylate remedies

Aspirin is a good simple painkiller and also has a high anti-inflammatory effect in rheumatism, provided high enough doses can be tolerated. Generally a dose of over 2.4 g of aspirin starts to produce side effects (*see* Chapter 16, pages 178–179).

Non-aspirin remedies

Active principal	Proprietary preparation	Dosage
Azapropazone	**Rheumox**	1.2 g daily, in two or four divided doses, after food

Table continued on next page

Non-aspirin remedies *continued*

Active principal	Proprietary preparation	Dosage
Diclofenac	Voltarol	25–50 mg thrice daily after meals; reduced if possible (rectally, 100 mg at night)
Diflunisal	(*See* Chapter 16, page 179)	
Fenbufen	Lederfen	600 mg daily as single dose at bedtime, or 600–900 mg daily in divided doses, after meals
Fenclofenac	Flenac	0.6–1.2 g daily in two divided doses, after meals; reduce to 900 mg per day
Fenoprofen	(*See* Chapter 16, page 180)	
Feprazone	Methrazone	200–600 mg daily in divided doses, after meals
Flufenamic acid	(*See* Chapter 16, page 180)	
Flurbiprofen	Froben	150–200 mg increased if necessary to 300 mg daily in three to four doses, after meals
Ibuprofen	Ibuprofen tablets Brufen Ebufac	200–400 mg thrice daily, after meals
Indoprofen	Flosint	200–600 mg daily in divided doses, with food
Ketoprofen	Ketoprofen capsules and suppository Alrheumat Orudis Oruvail	By mouth, 50 mg two to four times daily in divided doses, after food. 100 mg suppository used at night
Mefanamic acid	(*See* Chapter 16, page 180)	
Naproxen	(*See* Chapter 16, page 180)	
Piroxicam	Feldene	20 mg daily, increased to 40 mg if necessary
Sulindac	Clinoril	100–200 mg twice daily, after food
Tiaprofenic acid	Surgam	600 mg daily in divided doses, after food
Tolmetin	Tolectin Tolectin DS	0.6–1.8 g daily in divided doses, after meals

- *Basic precautions:* Not usually suitable if patient has a medical history of gastric ulcer, allergic diseases, particularly asthma (especially those sensitive to salicylates—aspirin). Also kidney or liver disease makes administration hazardous. Rectal suppositories not suitable if piles or proctitis are present. Feprazone not suitable in heart disease.
- *Proper dosage: See* table.
- *Side effects:* Mild gastric discomfort, sometimes gastric bleeding manifested as

dark-coloured vomit or black stools, allergic reactions, headache, dizziness, ringing in ears.
- *Special advantages:* Usually better tolerated than large doses of aspirin. Naproxen has lower incidence of side effects than most other remedies; it also has convenient twice daily dosage.

POWERFUL ANTI-INFLAMMATORY REMEDIES THAT MAY AFFECT THE RHEUMATIC PROCESS

These are often used when the remedies just detailed are found to be ineffective. Some of these drugs affect the disease process itself (rather than just alleviate symptoms). All are powerful and potentially dangerous but are highly effective if used properly and release many victims from suffering.

INDOMETHACIN

Artracin (capsules)
Imbrilon (capsules and suppositories)
Indocid (capsules, suspension and suppositories)
Indocid R (slow-release capsules)
Mobilan (capsules)
Osmosin (sustained release tablets)
Indomethacin (F) (capsules and suppositories)
- *Basic precautions:* Not suitable for patients with active peptic ulcer or a history of gastrointestinal upset, or if they are sensitive to aspirin. Care needed if driving or if work requires alertness and attention as dizziness may be a hazard. May aggravate epilepsy, psychiatric disorders, Parkinsonism. Regular ophthalmological supervision indicated. Not to be used in suppository form if piles or rectal bleeding are in evidence. If reactions occur, dosage should first be reduced and then, if necessary, stopped.
- *Proper usage:* The dosage and mode of use should be adjusted to individual patient's needs. Should be taken with food or milk, or an antacid should be taken after the dose of Indocid. Recommended starting dose of 50 mg per day, increasing to 200 mg per day if necessary. Suppository—1 to be used once or twice daily. Sustained release Indocid 'R' capsules—1 tablet once or twice daily. Osmosin—1 tablet, once or twice daily.
- *Side effects:* Headaches, dizziness, gastrointestinal upset, gastric ulcer, gastric haemorrhage, irritation of rectum when using suppositories. Because it has quite a powerful anti-inflammatory action, indomethacin may mask infection symptoms: a boil may be painless. Adverse reactions are more common in the elderly. Sensitivity reactions such as rashes, wheeziness are uncommon.
- *Special advantages:* Useful for treating a large number of rheumatic disorders. Very useful where sleep is disturbed by pain or morning stiffness is a feature of illness.

PHENYLBUTAZONE AND OXYPHENBUTAZONE

Tandacote (tablets)
Tanderil (tablets and suppositories)
Butacote (tablets)
Butazolidin (tablets and suppositories)

Butazolidin Alka (tablets)
Butazone (tablets)
Phenylbutazone (F) (tablets)

- *Basic precautions:* Not suitable if patients have high blood pressure, heart disease or heart failure (in which leg swelling is a common symptom). Not suitable in the presence of kidney or liver disease, history of peptic ulceration, blood diseases, drug rashes or sensitivities. Can potentiate some drugs used in diabetes. Blood counts before and during treatment recommended.
- *Proper usage:* Tablets—first two days, 400–600 mg daily in divided doses, with meals, followed by a sodium-free antacid (*see* Chapter 1). Dosage then reduced to 200–300 mg daily. Suppository—the equivalent of 250–500 mg daily.
- *Side effects:* Drug rashes, swelling of legs, vomiting of blood, swelling of saliva glands (like mumps), swelling of thyroid gland, jaundice occur rarely. Blood abnormalities may be caused, so blood count monitoring is essential.
- *Special advantages:* Relatively rare adverse effects have to be weighed against potent antirheumatic activity.

STEROIDS

See Chapter 2, pages 45–48 (Prednisolone is the drug usually used).

PENICILLAMINE

Cuprimine (capsules)
Distamine (tablets)
Pendramine (tablets)

- *Basic precautions:* Particular care should be exercised if the patient has a previous history of reaction to gold, or skin sensitivity reactions. Not to be given simultaneously with iron remedies. Routine blood and urine tests advisable.
- *Proper dosage:* Up to 250 mg daily for first four weeks, increasing by the amount of starting dose at intervals of four to eight weeks until symptoms regress. Dosage range—500 mg to 2 g daily, but can be variable. Response is slow (several weeks) so dose should be increased slowly to avoid unnecessary overdosage. Dose should be reduced at intervals of two to three months by 250 mg, to be taken daily to obtain effective maintenance.
- *Side effects:* These can usually be prevented by cautious dosage. Nausea, loss of appetite, vomiting, fever, rashes, spontaneous bruising; blood and kidney damage as evidenced by routine monitoring tests indicate that remedy should be withdrawn. Taste impairment may occur.
- *Special advantages:* A powerful drug similar to gold therapy (which is only given by injection under the supervision of a doctor).

CHLOROQUINE

Avloclor (tablets)
Malarivon (syrup)
Nivaquine (tablets, syrup and injection)
Plaquenil (tablets)

- *Basic precautions:* Not to be used if patient is sensitive to quinine or if drug that is potentially toxic to liver or gold therapy is being given.
- *Proper dosage:* Chloroquine—usually 150–300 mg daily, after meals, reduced to

150 mg daily when possible. Plaquenil—400–600 mg daily, reduced to 400 mg.
- *Side effects:* Gastrointestinal upset, headache, visual disturbances. Rare side effects may be irreversible damage to eyesight, loss of hair colour, loss of hair, rashes, dizziness, ringing in ears, deafness, muscle and nerve damage, psychiatric upsets, blood abnormalities.
- *Special advantages:* Despite potential dangers, these remedies help certain rare rheumatic diseases when others fail.

Treatment of gout

The management of gout falls into two stages: (1) treatment for the acute attack; and (2) remedies to prevent occurrence of further attacks.

ACUTE GOUT

Colchicine
Used as cover against attacks occurring while also taking preventative drugs.
- *Basic precautions:* To be used with care for the elderly or debilitated or those with heart disease, gastrointestinal or kidney disease. Not to be repeated within three days of previous use of drug.
- *Proper dosage:* 1 mg to be taken at first sign of attack, then 500 micrograms every two to three hours until relief of pain occurs or if vomiting or diarrhoea begins. Total dosage should not exceed 10 mg. Not to be repeated for three days. Taken as a preventative measure thereafter in first cases of the disease—500 micrograms, two to three times daily.

Naproxen (F), Indomethacin (F), Phenylbutazone (F)
(for naproxen *see* Chapter 16, page 180. For indomethacin and phenylbutazone, *see* this chapter, page 127)
- *Proper dosage:* Naproxen—750 mg initially then 250 mg eight-hourly. Indomethacin—50–100 mg repeated every three hours, frequency reduced to six-hourly as symptoms improve. Phenylbutazone—up to 800 mg per day.

PREVENTION OF CHRONIC ATTACKS

Gout is characterised by the accumulation of large quantities of uric acid in the body. There are two methods of combating this state to reduce or prevent the painful, damaging and repeated attacks of acute gout. First of all the formation of uric acid may be reduced by means of *inhibitor* drugs (allopurinol). Secondly, the excess of accumulated uric acid can be persuaded to leave the body by means of *uricosuric* drugs (probenecid, sulphinpyrazone). It is quite possible that the number of attacks of acute gout may increase during the first few months of preventative treatment unless 'cover' is given.

Inhibitor drugs

ALLOPURINOL
Zyloric
- *Basic precautions:* Not to be taken during an acute attack of gout.

- *Proper dosage:* 100–300 mg per day as single dose. If larger doses (up to 900 mg) are advised, should be taken in divided doses. Blood tests to monitor blood uric acid levels are essential—dosage is determined according to these results. Maintenance (continual) dose is usually 200–600 mg per day.
- *Side effects:* In an acute attack of gout, skin reactions may be caused by taking this medicine. If so, the drug should be withdrawn and cautiously reintroduced at 50 mg level. If rashes recur, treatment should be abandoned. Rare severe 'skinning'-type skin reactions (large patches of skin peeling) dictate immediate withdrawal of treatment. Rare gastrointestinal effects reported.
- *Special advantages:* Reduces blood uric acid to normal levels, thus preventing possibly dangerous effects of high levels on kidneys.

Uricosuric drugs

PROBENECID
Benemid
- *Basic precautions:* Not to be taken if patient has a previous history of blood diseases or if certain kidney stones have occurred. Not to be taken during, or within three weeks of, acute gout, or if salicylates (aspirin etc) are being taken. Special care if patients have peptic ulcer, kidney colic, blood in urine; special care if indomethacin is being taken. Not to be taken if kidney failure is suspected.
- *Side effects:* Mild hypersensitivity reactions (skin rashes and wheeziness).
- *Proper dosage:* 250 mg twice daily for one week, to be increased to 500 mg twice daily. Once satisfactory blood test levels for uric acid are obtained the dose should be reduced. The dosage at this stage is adjusted to produce an individual level of uric acid that is just tending to rise. Once blood uric acid is steady, dietary restrictions can be relaxed.
- *Special advantages:* Effective treatment.

SULPHINPYRAZONE
Anturan
- *Basic precautions:* Special care needed if patient has kidney disease or kidney stones. If diabetic remedies are being taken these may need reduction in dosage.
- *Proper dosage:* 100–200 mg daily as single dose, or divided, taken with meals or milk. Dosage is increased over two to three weeks to 600 mg daily until blood tests indicate reduction of dosage is possible. Reduced then to smallest maintenance dose (100–200 mg per day). Then continue indefinitely.
- *Side effects:* May cause acute gout attacks early on in treatment (increase intake of fluids and obtain alkalinisation of urine to counteract). Rare gastrointestinal bleeding, rashes, blood disorders (routine blood counts advised).
- *Special advantages:* Effective treatment.

Other treatments in rheumatism

In such a widespread disease, and one in which the natural history of the illness, and its sequelae, is so problematical, various and very variable treatments have gained credence. This does not mean that they are of dubious value: it is just that because rheumatism causes so much discomfort and disability there has been a propensity to espouse unorthodox and scientifically unproven treatment. Many such remedies have been found to be very helpful to sufferers. Some of these are listed below.

ENZYME TREATMENTS

These are suggested for soft tissue (non-articular) rheumatism.

BROMELAINS AND CHYMOTRYPSIN

Ananase Forte, Chymoral, Deanase DC

- *Basic precautions:* Care to be exercised if patient has blood clotting diseases, liver and kidney disease.
- *Proper dosage:* Ananase Forte—1 tablet four times daily. Chymoral—1 tablet four times daily, before meals. Deanase DC—2 tablets twice daily for three days, then 1 tablet twice daily.
- *Side effects:* Gastrointestinal symptoms, rashes and heavy menstrual periods.
- *Special advantages:* May be effective in a field where more conventional therapy is not notable for success.

COD LIVER OIL REMEDIES

Cod liver oil is manufactured mainly by one company which markets the Seven Seas range of products. For years now they have received many more testimonials (from people who take cod liver oil) referring to an improvement in a range of rheumatological conditions than would be expected. This is despite the fact that the product is not being primarily advertised as being beneficial for rheumatism. Unfortunately random double blind trials in this field are not possible and so attempts at understanding how this complex substance can help with rheumatism remain unanswered.

▲ Cod liver oil (F)

- *Basic precautions:* None.
- *Proper dosage:* 10 ml cod liver oil, twice daily.
- *Side effects:* None.
- *Special advantages:* Is effective in the management of many rheumatic symptoms.

▲ 'MUSSEL' CURES

Rheumatism therapy involving taking extracts from the cultivated New Zealand green-lipped mussel have been one of the most recent 'new' rheumatism treatments. Few scientific papers have supported the new therapy but enthusiastic reports have boosted sales.

Chapter

12

REMEDIES FOR NAUSEA AND GIDDINESS

It may seem odd that vomiting, sickness and giddiness (sometimes referred to by doctors as vertigo) should be lumped together as similar conditions. The logical explanation is that the two symptoms do sometimes occur together, or one after the other (motion can cause giddiness which is followed by vomiting). There is also an anatomical logic to this because the vomiting centre and the balance organ form adjacent areas in the brain. Although there is a considerable overlap therapeutically, in the remedies prescribed, it is convenient to consider these under the following headings:

Remedies for motion sickness and its treatment;
Remedies for pregnancy sickness;
Remedies for vomiting secondary to an illness;
Remedies for giddiness (vertigo).

Motion sickness and its treatment

There are two approaches to treatment with differing drugs. (1) *Anticholinergic drugs*—their action is detailed in Chapters 1 and 2. (2) *Antihistamines*—these drugs when first introduced were hailed as major therapeutic advances. Their name indicates that they tend to block the effect of a substance called *histamine*, one of the chemicals which promotes an allergic response when released into the bloodstream. As a result antihistamines were incorporated in medicines used where allergy seemed to play a large part in producing symptoms, eg the skin, the chest and the nose. Today they are much less used in this way, except perhaps in the nose (*see* Chapter 14). Antihistamines do, however, have a central effect on the brain and particularly the areas associated with motion sickness.

ANTICHOLINERGIC DRUGS

Active principal	Proprietary preparation	Formulary preparation
Atropine		Atropine sulphate tablets
Hyoscine	▲ Kwells, Sereen, Joyrides	Hyoscine tablets

- *Basic precautions:* Not suitable for glaucoma patients, those likely to be threatened with urinary retention (men with prostate problems); care advised in use for patients with heart disease. Should not be used concurrently with anti-depressants, particularly MAOIs.
- *Proper dosage:* Atropine tablets—0.25–2 mg daily or in single dose. Hyoscine tablets—300–600 micrograms four times daily. Take thirty minutes before travelling. Their short-acting effect lasts about six hours.
- *Side effects:* Drowsiness, dry mouth, blurred vision, difficulty in starting urination, rarely dizziness. May interfere with driving—so don't drive.
- *Special advantages:* Useful for short journeys.

ANTIHISTAMINE REMEDIES

Active principal	Proprietary preparation	
Cinnarizine	▲ Stugeron	
Cyclizine	▲ Valoid	▲ Marzine
Dimenhydrinate	▲ Dramamine	▲ Gravol
Diphenhydramine	▲ Benadryl	
Meclozine	▲ Ancoloxin	▲ Sealegs
Promethazine	▲ Phenergan	▲ Avomine

- *Basic precautions:* Reactions to antihistamines are somewhat unpredictable. Drowsiness occurs in many patients and can make driving hazardous. Alcohol potentiates these effects.
- *Proper dosage:* Cinnarizine—15–30 mg thrice daily two hours before start of journey. Cyclizine remedies—50 mg thrice daily. Dimenhydrinate—50–100 mg three times daily; maximum dosage 300 mg daily. Suppository—100 mg up to four times daily. Diphenhydramine remedies—25–50 mg three to four times daily. Meclozine—25–50 mg up to thrice daily. Promethazine—25–75 mg per day in single or divided dosage.
- *Side effects:* Drowsiness, aftertaste in mouth, dry mouth.
- *Special advantages:* Long-acting remedies—the suppository form is often an advantage in sea-sickness.

Pregnancy sickness and its treatment

The consensus of medical opinion holds that remedies used to treat pregnancy sickness are not entirely without risk, and doctors prefer not to use any anti-nausea remedies unless vomiting is a major problem.

Vomiting secondary to illness

This can range from a bilious attack, or an attack of gastroenteritis, to drug-induced vomiting or post-irradiation vomiting. Often in such cases the rectal administration of the drug by suppository is advisable. Excess loss of body fluids should be remedied by the use of Dioralyte (*see* page 27).

Preparations commonly used
See also antihistamines, previous pages.

CHLORPROMAZINE
Largactil
- *Basic precautions:* Care advised in use for patients with heart and blood vessel disease, Parkinsonism, epilepsy, kidney or liver disease, especially jaundice. However, these considerations still allow occasional use in small doses. May cause drowsiness so driving and machinery operation can be a hazard.
- *Proper dosage:* 25–50 mg thrice daily. Suppository—100 mg thrice daily.
- *Side effects:* Drowsiness, nightmares, apathy, depression of mood—even at quite low doses.
- *Special advantages:* Useful and potent antivomiting remedy, especially in suppository form.

METOCLOPRAMIDE
Maxolon
- *Basic precautions:* None for occasional use.
- *Proper dosage:* 10 mg thrice daily.
- *Side effects:* In prolonged use there can be increased muscle tone and tension, spasm of face muscles and an unnatural positioning of head on shoulders.
- *Special advantages:* Restores normal passage of contents of stomach into the bowel. A useful addition to available remedies.

Dizziness (giddiness, vertigo)

Vertigo is characterised by a person feeling a sensation of movement in the environment when in fact this is not actually happening. It seems to the victim as if everything around him is spinning, rising or sinking. Often sweating, pallor, nausea and vomiting complicate the symptom. Vertigo can be caused in many ways. Two common causes are infection of the balance organ in the ear (labyrinthitis) or a disease of the inner ear called Ménière's disease. It can also occur after ear and brain surgery. Treatment includes all the previous antivomiting remedies, together with certain rather more specific remedies. These vary in effectiveness, sometimes mitigating only certain systems, as in the case of the tinnitus (ringing in the ears) of Ménière's disease.

Preparations commonly used

PROCHLORPERAZINE
Stemetil, Vertigon
- *Basic precautions:* Not suitable for patients with liver damage or blood diseases. Care to be exercised in use by elderly or those with heart disease. May cause sudden lowering of blood pressure, also 'peaking' and 'troughing', dizziness and collapse. Drowsiness may preclude safe driving and machinery operation.
- *Proper dosage:* Stemetil 5 mg tablets—4 tablets followed by 2 tablets two hours later if necessary for vomiting; otherwise 5 mg thrice daily. Suppositories—25 mg once or twice daily. Vertigon slow-release capsules (spansules)—two

strengths (10 and 15 mg). Usual dosage 15 mg capsule once or twice daily; if symptoms are less severe the 10 mg once or twice daily.

• *Side effects:* Drowsiness, dizziness, rashes, dry mouth.

• *Special advantages:* Useful for short-term therapy. Long-term less advisable because of effects on coordination.

BUCLIZINE (WITH NICOTINIC ACID)

Equivert

• *Basic precautions:* Drowsiness may preclude safe driving and machinery operation.

• *Proper dosage:* 25 mg thrice daily before meals.

• *Side effects:* Short-lived skin flushing and tingling sensations. Increased bowel movements, greasy skin, drowsiness, headache and rare dryness of mouth.

• *Special advantages:* Useful for treating vertigo generally, whatever the cause.

BETAHISTINE

Serc

• *Basic precautions:* Not to be taken if patient has the fairly rare disease phaeochromocytoma.

• *Proper dosage:* 8 mg tablet—1–2 tablets thrice daily after meals; maximum dosage 48 mg per day.

• *Side effects:* Rare gastric upset.

• *Special advantages:* Claimed as a specific remedy for Ménière's disease.

THIETHYLPERAZINE

Torecan

• *Basic precautions:* Not suitable for severely depressed patients. Use may impair the amount of time required for reaction to situations.

• *Proper dosage:* Tablets—1 tablet two to three times daily. Suppositories—1 night and morning.

• *Side effects:* Potentiates action of alcohol. Drowsiness, dryness of mouth, mental depression.

• *Special advantages:* Controls vomiting and vertigo. Useful for all problems associated with these symptoms.

Chapter

13

REMEDIES THAT ACT ON THE EYE

Most of us worry about the health of our eyes and no wonder, because vision is an extremely valuable thing. Remedies for eye problems are seldom self-administered and selected, and when they are, often they are potentially hazardous (for example mercuric oxide, 'Golden Eye Ointment') and are unlikely to help the symptoms that occasion their use. For instance, there are still proprietary eye lotions advertised to help with 'tired eyes' and the like, when it has been repeatedly pointed out by ophthalmic specialists that, in fact, eyes do not 'tire' in this way. There are, however, special problems involved in patients with reduced tear secretion.

Eye remedies fall into the following groups:

Remedies to combat local infection in or around the eye;

Remedies used to treat allergic problems involving the conjunctiva (the 'skin' over the eyeball);

Remedies for the treatment of specific eye diseases, particularly corneal ulceration and glaucoma.

Remedies used to combat infection

Most medicines administered in the form of eye-drops or ointments not only act on the conjunctiva covering the eyeball they also penetrate the eyeball itself. They can be absorbed to some extent into the general circulation via the conjunctiva, or through the nasal passages that drain away the eye's tears into the nose. The extent to which this occurs is not necessarily small—enough *beta*-blocking action occurs after the use of timolol eye-drops to slow the pulse rate. Sometimes this unsuspected ability of the humble eye-drop to change things has to be taken into account by user and doctor.

Generally speaking, eye-drops, because they are soon diluted by the tears, have a less marked action than eye ointments. It is important that eye-drops and oint-ments should not be contaminated before use. Most contain a suitable preservative, and provided they are carefully used, can function safely for about one month, although patients should always examine labels for expiry dates. After this a new pack should always be used and old preparations discarded.

Eye ointments usually only need to be applied every three to four hours—drops often more frequently, especially in acute infection.

REMEDIES FOR EYE INFECTIONS

Available as eye-drops and eye ointment, unless specified in other form.

Active principal	Proprietary preparation		Formulary preparation
Acyclovir	Zovirax	(ointment only)	
Chloramphenicol	Chloromycetin Minims chloramphenicol Sno-Phenicol		Chloramphenicol
Chlortetracycline	Aureomycin	(ointment only)	
Dibromopropamidine	▲ Brolene		
Framycetin	Framygen Soframycin		
Gentamicin	Genticin		
Idoxuridine	Dendrid Idoxene Kerecid Ophthalmadine	(drops only) (ointment only)	Idoxuridine
Mafenide	▲ Sulfomyl	(drops only)	
Neomycin/gramicidin	Graneodin Minims neomycin sulphate Myciguent	(ointment only) (drops only) (ointment only)	
Polymixin B sulphate	Polyfax	(ointment only)	
Sulphacetamide	Albucid Bleph-10 liquifilm Isopto cetamide Minims sulphacetamide Ocusol	 (drops only) (drops only) (drops only) (drops only)	
Tetracycline	Achromycin		
Trimethoprim	Polytrim	(drops only)	
Vidarabine	Vira-A	(ointment only)	

Eye-drops—general application

The following cautions apply to all of the above drugs with the exception of acyclovir and idoxuridine preparations, and Graneodin, a derivative of neomycin/gramicidin.

- *Basic precautions:* Make sure preparation is within the date of use. Not to be used if patient is known to be sensitive to active principal.
- *Proper usage:* When eye-drops are being used to combat infection, ideally they should be instilled into the eye every ten minutes or so for the first hour, and then hourly for the first day or so. To effectively place drops into the eye, it is best to lie on your back and lift the upper lid off the eyeball, allowing the dropper to deposit the drops in the space between the lid and the eyeball.

- *Side effects:* The possibility of secondary infection with fungus and organisms that are not sensitive to the drops must be borne in mind. Any signs of reinfection or exacerbation of symptoms should be reported to doctor.

Special exceptions—(acyclovir and idoxuridine)

The antiviral preparations (acyclovir and idoxuridine) have to be used with particular caution, especially when being used for herpes virus infection. Such eyedrops should not be used if patients are taking steroids, whether by mouth or by aerosols and topical preparations.

ACYCLOVIR
Zovirax

A one-centimetre length of ointment squeezed from tube should be placed on the space between lower eyelid and eye five times daily, at four-hourly intervals. Continue for at least three days after apparent cure.

IDOXURIDINE
Dendrid, Idoxene, Kerecid, Ophthalmadine and Idoxuridine preparations (F)

1 drop used hourly during day and two-hourly at night until inflamed area does not stain; then two-hourly by day and four-hourly at night for a further three to five days. Maximum length of treatment twenty-one days.

NEOMYCIN/GRAMICIDIN

- *Basic precautions:* Not to be used in virus or fungal infections.

Steroid preparations

These are used to treat various specific eye diseases and are very effective in action. There are some potential problems that, although rare, are serious when encountered. An increasingly prevalent eye inflammation is that caused by herpes simplex virus which often produces a special type of corneal ulcer. Steroids, with or without the antibiotics that these preparations may contain, can encourage such eye ulcers to enlarge, and loss of vision and/or loss of eyes themselves have occurred. Thus, when such preparations are prescribed the strictest medical supervision is mandatory. There is a further hazard in using these otherwise excellent preparations. Many patients suffer from the disease known as simple glaucoma— often undiagnosed in its early stages. After a week's treatment with local steroids the eyes may react by passing into an acute steroid-induced glaucoma with a subsequent acute threat to vision.

'SIMPLE' STEROID PREPARATIONS

Active principal	Proprietary preparation
Betamethasone	Betnesol
Clobetasone	Eumovete
Dexamethasone	Maxidex
Fluorometholone	FML Liquifilm
Prednisolone	Predsol

• *Basic precautions, side effects, etc:* Since all these preparations are—or should be—administered under the strictest control of a doctor, and the precautions and side effects vary considerably according to the condition being treated, no general guidelines can be given. But when the drug and disease have been well matched, the success rate is impressive. Steroids reduce the body's immulogical response to bacterial and other infections, and so antibiotics are often prescribed concurrently.

MIXED PREPARATIONS (including steroids with antibiotics)

To the general hazards of the steroids in eye-drops must be added the potential sensitivity hazards of the various antibiotics and other anti-inflammatory compounds that they contain.

Proprietary preparations	Principal components
Betresol-N eye drops and eye ointment	Betamethasone, neomycin
Chloromycetin Hydrocortisone eye ointment	Chloramphenicol, hydrocortisone acetate
Cortucid eye-drop cream	Hydrocortisone acetate, sulphacetamide sodium
Eumovate-N eye drops	Clobetasone, neomycin
Framycort (for ear or eye)	Framycetin sulphate, hydrocortisone acetate
Maxitrol eye-drops	Dexamethasone, hypromellose, neomycin sulphate, polymyxin B sulphate
eye ointment	Ingredients as for eye-drops, except for hypromellose
Neo-Cortef drops and ointment	Hydrocortisone and neomycin
Neosporin eye-drops	Gramicidin, neomycin sulphate, polymyxin B sulphate
Ocusol eye-drops	Sulphacetamide sodium, zinc sulphate
▲ **Otrivine-Antistin** eye-drops	Antazoline sulphate, xylometazoline hydrochloride
Polyfax eye ointment	Bacitracin zinc, polymyxin B sulphate
Predsol-N eye drops	Prednisolone, neomycin
Sulfapred eye-drops	Prednisolone sodium, m-sulphobenzoate, sulphacetamide sodium
Tanderil/Chloramphenicol eye ointment	Chloramphenicol, oxyphenbutazone
Terramycin Ophthalmic Ointment with Polymyxin B Sulphate eye ointment	Oxytetracycline hydrochloride, polymyxin B sulphate
Vasocon A eye drops	Naphazoline and antazoline
▲ **Zincfrin** eye-drops	Phenylephrine hydrochloride, zinc sulphate

• *Basic precautions:* Not suitable for some contact lens users (consult optician), or for glaucoma sufferers, in inflammatory conditions in which virus, pus-forming or tuberculous infection is suspected, or if cataracts are present. Preparations not to be used for prolonged periods. Not to be used if known sensitivity to antibiotic.
• *Proper usage:* 1–2 drops used every one to two hours until control is achieved,

then reduce dosage. In case of ointments a quarter-inch-long strip of tube contents are applied to inside lower eyelid two to three times daily and at night.

- *Side effects:* Induced glaucoma, cataract, thinning and possible perforation of cornea, extension of herpetic ulceration.
- *Special advantages:* Used with proper care and supervision these products can cure a large number of otherwise intractable eye conditions.

Other eye-drops for inflammation and allergy

In a bid to provide less hazardous preparations to combat infection and allergy in the eye, other products have been developed.

PRESCRIPTION-ONLY REMEDIES

OXYPHENBUTAZONE

Tanderil (eye ointment)

Tanderil/Chloramphenicol (eye ointment)

- *Basic precautions:* None.
- *Proper usage:* Use a quarter-inch-long strip of ointment on the inside eyelid two to five times daily.
- *Side effects:* Rare sensitivity.
- *Special advantages:* Useful and safe remedy.

SODIUM CROMOGLYCATE

Opticrom (eye-drops)

- *Basic precautions:* None.
- *Proper usage:* 1–2 drops in each eye four times daily.
- *Side effects:* None.
- *Special advantages:* Useful preparation that works by the process of mast cell stabilisation.

OTC REMEDIES

Proprietary preparation	Principal components
▲ Mercuric Oxide	Eye ointment, mercuric oxide—an old-fashioned and largely outmoded remedy commonly called 'Golden Eye Ointment'
▲ Clearine Eye-Drops	Witch hazel, naphazoline
▲ Eye Dew Eye-Drops	Witch hazel, naphazoline
▲ Murine Eye-Drops	Naphazoline and boric acid
▲ Optabs Eye Lotion Solution Tablets	Adrenaline, phenylephrine, acriflavine
▲ Optrex Drops	Witch hazel, allantoin, chlorbutol
▲ Optrex Eye Ointment	Gramiciden, aminacrine
▲ Optrex Eye Lotion	Witch hazel, allantoin, salicylic acid, chlorbutol, zinc sulphate

These are widely-used OTC remedies which have produced few side effects, if used as recommended by the manufacturers.

The management of glaucoma

The management of glaucoma is best regulated by a glaucoma clinic. The most efficient of these work in conjunction with a computerised patient management and data recall system, so that the indications for changes in treatment may be accurately logged and patients' stability in treatment maintained. Generally speaking, the aim of treatment is to reduce pressure inside the eyeball by means of medicines taken by mouth or by the use of eye-drops. Often a combination of treatments is necessary and sometimes changes in formulation or strengths of drops must be made to ensure good pressure control and thus stabilise vision which otherwise deteriorates.

TREATMENT BY TABLETS

ACETAZOLAMIDE
Diamox, Diamox Sustets

- *Basic precautions:* Not suitable for patients with certain kidney diseases, Addison's disease (or other adrenal diseases), chronic non-congestive angle-closure glaucoma, or if skin rashes develop. Periodic blood counts are necessary in long-term treatment. Should hearing loss occur, immediate cessation of treatment is advised. Caution is also advised in patients taking lithium salts or certain medications for heart disease.
- *Proper dosage:* 1–4 tablets daily. Sustets—1 capsule night and morning.
- *Side effects:* Drowsiness, pins and needles, gastrointestinal upsets, flushing, thirst, frequent urine passing, headache, dizziness, irritability, depression; more rarely fever, anaemia, kidney stone problems and occasionally short-sightedness develops.
- *Special advantages:* For suitable cases a valuable aid to glaucoma control.

DICHLORPHENAMIDE
Daranide, Oratrol

- *Basic precautions:* Not suitable for patients with liver disease, kidney failure, adrenal disease, or severe lung disease.
- *Proper dosage:* Initially 2–4 tablets followed by 2 tablets twelve-hourly. Maintenance dosage—$\frac{1}{2}$–1 tablet one to three times daily.
- *Side effects:* Gastrointestinal upset, loss of weight, constipation, frequent urine passing, thirst, development of kidney stones, headaches, weakness, drowsiness, unsteadiness, ringing in ears, pins and needles, depression.
- *Special advantages:* As for acetazolamide. Also has a more prolonged action.

TREATMENT BY DROPS

Most of these drops act by producing a small pupil. This reduction in pupil size tends to open up inefficient drainage channels within the eye, which seems to be the fundamental cause of glaucoma. Management usually evolves around using the weakest type of drop that will be compatible with reducing the internal pressure inside the eyeball to a level which prevents any further deterioration of vision occurring. An ophthalmic surgeon usually dictates treatment and strengths of drops.

ADRENALINE
Epifrin, Simplene
▲ Eppy, Isopto Epinal
- *Basic precautions:* Not to be used to treat narrow-angle glaucoma.
- *Proper usage:* 1 drop in eye once or twice daily. Discard after one month of opening.
- *Side effects:* Red, sore eyes, palpitation.
- *Special advantages:* Does not affect accommodation (focusing of eyes).

DEMECARIUM
Tosmilen
- *Basic precautions:* Not to be used by asthmatics or bronchitics; not to be used for patients with gastric or duodenal ulcer or if a patient's pulse is very slow.
- *Proper usage:* 1–2 drops two or three times daily.
- *Side effects:* Red, sore eyes.
- *Special advantages:* Useful for treating chronic primary glaucoma.

ECOTHIOPATE
Phospholine Iodine
- *Basic precautions:* Not to be used to treat closed-angle glaucoma, certain eye inflammations or patients with asthma.
- *Proper usage:* 1–2 drops night and morning.
- *Side effects:* 'Brow' headache, red eyes, blurred vision (especially to start with), lens opacities (cataract), rarely cysts in iris.
- *Special advantages:* Less frequent dosage makes use easier.

GUANETHIDINE REMEDIES
Ganda, Ismelin
- *Basic precautions:* Not to be used to treat narrow-angle glaucoma. Not to be used if discoloration of drops occurs.
- *Proper usage:* 1 drop once or twice daily.
- *Side effects:* Red eye, headache, palpitation.
- *Special advantages:* Less frequent dosage makes use easier.

PHYSOSTIGMINE AND PILOCARPINE REMEDIES
Isopto-Carpine, Ocusert, Sno Pilo, Minims Pilocarpine Nitrate, Physostigmine (F), Pilocarpine (F) and Physostigmine and Pilocarpine drops (F)
- *Basic precautions:* These drops contract the pupil, and so should not be used in conditions where it is incompatible with treatment.
- *Proper usage:* 1–2 drops four times daily.
- *Side effects:* Red eye, headache, 'darkening' of vision, poor night vision. Rare cases of sensitivity, blurring of vision.
- *Special advantages:* Effective and safe remedy.

TIMOLOL
Timoptol

- *Basic precautions:* Not to be used for patients with asthma, slow pulse, heart disease.
- *Proper usage:* 1 drop twice daily.
- *Side effects:* Rare dry eyes.
- *Special advantages:* A very effective drug, with general freedom from side effects.

Other eye problems

REMEDIES FOR EXCESSIVE TEARS

One problem connected with eyes is that of excessive production of tears. An apparent excess of tears is often due in fact to an obstruction of the tear drainage system and a simple operation may be beneficial.

▲ **Zinc sulphate** drops are astringent and are traditionally used to reduce the amount of tears.

▲ **Zinc and Adrenaline** drops should not be used if there is any risk of the patient having closed-angle glaucoma, though otherwise the dilation of pupil helps to drain the tear ducts.

REMEDIES FOR TEARLESS EYES

A deficient supply of tears sometimes needs to be treated. This condition may be an annoying accompaniment to rheumatoid arthritis. Hypromellose drops are often prescribed as are Liquifilm Tears.

HYPROMELLOSE EYE DROPS
▲ Isopto Alkaline, Isopto Plain, Tears Naturale

- *Basic precautions:* Not suitable for soft contact lens users.
- *Proper usage:* 1–2 drops thrice daily, or more frequently if necessary. To preserve sterility of solution do not allow dropper to touch lashes or eyelid.
- *Side effects:* None.
- *Special advantages:* Effective supplier of artificial tears.

POLYVINYL ALCOHOL
▲ Liquifilm Tears

As for hydromellose preparations.

14

THE PROBLEMS OF THE EAR, NOSE, MOUTH AND THROAT AND THEIR TREATMENT

The ear

Though the ear may be affected by the common cold and flu, there are three basic problems which are more particular to the organ—impaired hearing due to accumulation of wax; the skin condition of otitis; and infection of the middle ear.

WAX IN THE EAR

Perhaps the most common problem relating to the ear is dealing with wax. A certain amount of wax in the ear is healthy: it is protective (common opinion holds that it prevents creepy crawlies entering the ear), and it 'waterproofs' the external ear (when the head is submerged). Ear wax in certain people, however, tends to accumulate and causes deafness, discomfort, and if it leads to ears being picked-at, sometimes infection or injury to the eardrum. And so wax-removing agents have a validity and are frequently prescribed.

The common preparations for dealing with wax

▲ **Sodium bicarbonate drops (F)**
▲ **Olive oil (F)**
▲ **Glycerol (F)**
   ● *Proper usage:* These preparations should be applied to a firm, well-wrapped plug of cotton wool which should be allowed to stay in the ear overnight for three nights. This generally allows wax to fall off the eardrum and sides of the ear from whence it finds its way out externally. If not, wax must be syringed out by a doctor or experienced nurse.

More sophisticated preparations
Used according to manufacturers' instructions.

▲ **Audinorm, Cerumol, Exterol, Molcer, Soliwax, Waxsol, Xerumenex, Product Earax**
   ● *Side effects:* Cerumol and Xerumenex can cause local irritation in rare cases.

OTITIS

This is a skin condition involving the 'hidden' skin inside the ear. Or it may involve the external part of the ear (*otitis externa*). If ear wax is present this can compound the problem which is usually manifested by a mildly sore ear which discharges constantly. Some cases of *otitis externa* need repeated *aural toilet* by an experienced ear, nose and throat surgeon to bring about a cure. But drops and ear ointments are often all that is necessary.

Simple remedies—ointments and ear drops

Active principal	Proprietary preparation	Formulary preparation
Aluminium acetate		▲ Aluminium Acetate ear drops
Betamethasone (steroid)	Betnesol	
Chloramphenicol	Chloromycetin Otopred	Chloramphenicol ear drops
Clioquinol	Locorten-Vioform	
Framycetin	Framygen	
Framycetin with steroid	Framycort	
Gentamicin	Genticin	
Gentamicin with hydrocortisone	Gentisone HC	
Halquinol with steroid	Remotic	
Neomycin with steroid	Audicort Betnesol-N Neo-cortef Predsol-N	
Prednisolone (steroid)	Predsol	
Tetracycline	Achromycin	

(For details of use, *see* Appendix, pages 193–195.)

Compound preparations—ointments and drops

In this field many 'mixed' preparations are popular. Sometimes they are helpful in cases of simple *otitis externa*. But they are also prescribed when pain in the ear indicates that a middle ear infection *otitis media* is present. *Otitis media* always needs medical management, and if a discharge follows an acutely painful ear (earache) then the chances are that the eardrum has been ruptured and a mixture of mucus and pus is finding its way to the exterior. A doctor should always be consulted in such cases.

It is often quite difficult to decide which ingredient is intended to be the main therapeutic agent in these remedies. These are generally steroids, antibiotics and bacteriocidal preparations.

Proprietary preparation	Main ingredients
▲ Audax	Choline/macrogol

Table continued on next page

Compound preparations *continued*

Proprietary preparation	Main ingredients
Audicort	Steroid/neomycin/benzocaine
▲ Auralgicin	Ephedrine/benzocaine
▲ Auraltone	Phenazone/benzocaine
▲ Norgotin	Ephedrine/amethocaine
Otoseptil	Steroid/neomycin
Otosporin	Polymyxin B/steroid/neomycin
Ototrips	Polymyxin B/bacitracin
▲ Sedonan	Phenazone/chlorbutol
Sofradex	Steroid/framycetin
Soframycin	Framycetin/gramicidin
Terra-Cortril	Oxytetracycline/steroid
Tri-Adcortyl Otic	Steroid/neomycin/gramicidin/nystatin

● *Basic precautions:* Framycetin, gentamycin, neomycin must not be used if eardrum is perforated. The various compounds (steroids and antibiotics and bacteriocidal preparations) used in the ear remedies are really acting primarily as they do on skin. Read this section, therefore, in conjunction with Chapter 10. As the skin area for steroid absorption is small, however, the various warnings concerning the adverse affects of most steroids can be discounted for internal ear treatment.

● *Proper usage:* First clear ear canal with cotton wool buds until bud emerges unstained. Do not push bud deeply into ear or use loose cotton wool in ear. Ointment or drops—3–4 drops thrice daily.

● *Side effects:* Consult the doctor immediately if there is any pain, stinging or bleeding. Skin reactions are possible with many local anaesthetics (benzocaine, amethocaine). Chloramphenicol used in the ear quite commonly causes local irritation, and in rare cases, deafness.

● *Special advantages:* Fungal infections in the ear often follow the use of antibiotics or antibacterial preparations. Then nystatin, clioquinol or neomycin preparations are useful.

The nose

There are several main areas of treatment: (1) for colds; (2) for nasal allergy; (3) for shrinking the nasal mucous membrane to allow sinuses to be better aerated; and (4) sinus infection.

Colds and nasal allergy are so similar in their local symptomatology that they can conveniently be dealt with together although their causes are vastly different. Colds are 'treated' (if this is the right word) in many ways; with vitamin C and with painkillers (*see* pages 177–181) and proprietary cold and cough medicines (*see* pages 49–52). From the practical point of view the remedies for nose problems might sensibly be considered as *remedies for the streaming or the obstructed (congested) nose.* When sinuses, tonsils or naso-pharynx tract generally are infected, then treatment for infection is necessary.

REMEDIES FOR THE OBSTRUCTED NOSE

Many nasal drops relieve congestion quickly, notably those using *sympathomimetic* drugs (*see* ephedrine, page 42). Unfortunately a 'rebound' effect (the patient becoming better, but then somewhat worse) tends to limit their usefulness and also leads, in many cases, to dependence. With prolonged use there can be damage to the nose's self-clearing action by its *cilia*. In many cases the misuse of nasal drops or ointments causes more problems than are solved.

Nose drops and sprays requiring special care

Active principal	Proprietary preparation	Formulary preparation
Ephedrine and derivatives	▲ Argotone Biomydrin* ▲ Fenox ▲ Hayphryn ▲ Neophryn Rhinamid* Soframycin* Vibrocil*	Ephedrine nasal drops
Metazoline derivatives	▲ Afrazine ▲ Antistin-Privine ▲ Dristan Nasal Mist ▲ Iliadin ▲ Otrivine ▲ Vicks Sinex Drops and Spray	
Cromoglycate	▲ Lomusol ▲ Rynacrom	
Steroid preparations	Beconase Betnesol Betnesol-N* Dexa-Rhinaspray* Syntaris	

* Also contains antibiotic/other ingredients.

- *Basic precautions:* Both ephedrine and metazoline preparations should be used with care in patients with heart disease, hypertension, palpitation. Secondary nasal congestion (rebound congestion) is common. Ephedrine and metazoline preparations should also not be used in conjunction with MAOI drugs (*see* Chapter 15, pages 164–167). Beware the rapid development of dependence. Steroid preparations should not be used if the patient has an infection, and caution must be exercised if the patient is on other steroids. Antibiotic preparations* should not be used if the patient has been shown to be sensitive to antibiotics in the past.
- *Proper usage:* Use three times daily—the exact mode of use should be according to manufacturer's instructions.
- *Side effects: See* basic precautions. Ephedrine has also been shown to cause headaches and excitement of the central nervous system.
- *Special advantages:* Cromoglycate has a special antiallergic effect. Steroid preparations are especially useful for short usage and if nasal symptoms tend to lead on to chest problems in any particular patient.

Sprays, drops and ointments without sympathomimetic drugs

Proprietary preparation	Ingredients
▲ Karvol Inhalant Capsules	Chlorbutanol, cinnamon, pine oils, terpineol, thymol
▲ Penetrol Inhalant	Menthol, cajuput, lavender, eucalyptus and peppermint oils
▲ Mentholatum Balm	Camphor, boric acid, eucalyptus and pine oils, methyl salicylate
▲ Olbas Oil	Cajuput, clove, eucalyptus, juniper and peppermint oils, menthol, wintergreen
▲ Vapex Inhalant	Menthol, eucalyptus, lavender and camphor oils
▲ Vicks Inhaler	Menthol, camphor, pine oil, methyl salicylate
▲ Vicks Vaporub	Eucalyptus, nutmeg, cedar wood and turpentine oils, menthol, camphor and thymol

The above preparations need no special precautions and cause no disturbing side effects if used according to the manufacturer's instructions.

TABLETS AND CAPSULES FOR THE STREAMING NOSE

These include *sympathomimetic* drugs (*see* Bronchodilators, page 38), *antihistamines* (*see* pages 132–133) and the specific antiallergic cromoglycate drugs. The last are generally applied locally in the nose. Steroid tablets are used very occasionally (*see* Chapter 2, pages 45–48).

Active principal	Proprietary preparation	Proper dosage
Sympathomimetics *Those drugs which also contain antihistamines	▲ Actifed*	1 tablet thrice daily
	▲ Benafed*	5 ml four times daily
	▲ Dimotapp*	1–2 tablets twice daily
	▲ Dimotapp P*	1–2 tablets thrice daily
	▲ Dimotapp LA	1–2 tablets night and morning
	▲ Eskornade*	Capsule—1 twice daily. Syrup—10 ml thrice daily
	▲ Histalix*	5–10 ml three-hourly
	▲ Paragesic	1–2 tablets four-hourly
	▲ Rinurel	2 tablets initially, then 1 four-hourly (maximum 6 in twenty-four hours)
	Rinurel SA	1 tablet twelve-hourly
	▲ Sudafed	1 tablet three times daily
	▲ Sudafed CO	1 tablet three times daily
	▲ Triocos*	10 ml thrice daily
	▲ Triogesic	1–2 tablets thrice daily
	▲ Triominic*	1 tablet six-hourly
	▲ Triotussic*	5–10 ml four-hourly
	▲ Uniflu + Gregovite C*	1 tablet of each four-hourly (maximum 6 in twenty-four hours)
	Vallex*	5–10 ml thrice daily

Antihistamines		
Azatadine	▲ Optimine	Tablets—1–2 twice daily. Syrup—10–20 ml twice daily
Brompheniramine	▲ Dimotane	1–2 tablets thrice daily
	▲ Dimotane LA	1–2 tablets twelve-hourly
Chlorpheniramine	▲ Haymine	1 tablet one to two times daily
	▲ Piriton	Tablets—1 thrice daily. Syrup—10 ml thrice daily. Spandets—1 twelve-hourly
Clemastine	Tavegil	1 tablet or 10 ml syrup twice daily
Cyproheptadine	▲ Periactin	Tablets—1 four times daily. Syrup—10 ml four times daily
Dimethindene	▲ Fenostil Retard	1 tablet night and morning
Dimethothiazine	Banistyl	1 tablet thrice daily
Diphenhydramine	▲ Benadryl	1 capsule thrice daily
Diphenylpyraline	▲ Histryl	1 tablet night and morning
	▲ Lergoban	1–2 tablets twelve-hourly
Mebhydrolin	▲ Fabahistin	1–2 tablets thrice daily
Mepyramine	▲ Anthisan	1 tablet thrice daily
Mequitazine	Primalan	1 tablet twice daily
Oxatomide	Tinset	1–2 twice daily after food
Phenindamine	▲ Thephorin	1–2 tablets thrice daily, last dose before 4 pm
Pheniramine	▲ Daneral SA	1–2 tablets at night, or 1 night and morning
Promethazine	▲ Phenergan	10–25 mg thrice daily. Elixir—10–20 ml thrice daily
Terfenadine	Triludan	1 tablet twice daily
Triprolidine	Actidil	Tablets—1–2 twice daily or elixir—5–10 ml thrice daily
	Pro-Actidil	1 tablet daily, five hours before bedtime

- *Basic precautions and side effects:* These have to take into account the sympatho-mimetic and antihistamine functions of the drugs (*see* Chapters 2 and 12). Thus, patients with glaucoma, prostate gland, thyroid and blood pressure problems, as well as coronary disease, diabetic and hypertensive disease patients, should ask if they can take any sympathomimetic drug. Such remedies should not be taken during or within two weeks of MAOI therapy (*see* pages 164–166). Anti-histamines may cause drowsiness and should not be used by drivers or those operating machinery. Certain drugs and alcohol can potentiate all antihistamines and make them much more sedating.
- *Special advantages:* Night-time dosage schedules are particularly useful. Thephorin is not sedative in its action in most people.

General flu remedies

Generally speaking, the preparations below may soothe and anaesthetise the nose and throat, through the action of salts, oils or ascorbic acid, and may supply a certain amount of decongestant aid. But they provide only symptom relief—in varying degrees—and can do nothing to alleviate the basic viral cause of the flu.

Proprietary preparation	Components
▲ Beecham's Powders, Mentholated	Aspirin, caffeine, menthol
▲ Beecham's Powders, Hot Lemon	Aspirin, caffeine, ascorbic acid, lemon, cinnamon
▲ Benylin Day and Night	Day tablets: Paracetamol, phenylpropanolamine Night tablets: Paracetamol, diphenhydramine
▲ Contac 400 Capsules	Phenylpropanolamine, belladonna
▲ Day Nurse	Paracetamol, vitamin C, phenylpropanolamine, dextramethorphan
▲ Dristan Tablets	Phenylephrine, chlorpheniramine, aspirin, caffeine
▲ Coldrex Tablets	Paracetamol, phenylephrine, caffeine, terpin, ascorbic acid
▲ Lemsip Sachets	Paracetamol, phenylephrine, sodium citrate, ascorbic acid, lemon
▲ Mucron Tablets	Guaiphenesin, phenylpropanolamine, ipecacuana, paracetamol
▲ Mucron Children's Liquid	Phenylpropanolamine, guaiphenesin
▲ Night Nurse	Promethazine, dextromethorphan, paracetamol
▲ Potter's Catarrh Pastilles	Pine and eucalyptus oils, creosote, menthol, thymol
▲ Procol Capsules	Isopropamide, phenylpropanolamine
▲ Sine-Off Tablets	Aspirin, phenylpropanolamine, chlorpheniramine
▲ Vicks Medinite	Dextromethorphan, ephedrine, doxylamine, paracetamol

General mouth and throat problems

While there are relatively few really useful preparations used medically for the mouth and throat, proprietary preparations and OTC remedies abound. There is probably no other area in which what the doctors feel is necessary, and what patients ask for in treatment, differ so radically. Throat lozenges and gargles, although widely prescribed and purchased, often seem to produce more problems than they solve. Acute infections of the throat often need the appropriate antibacterial or antibiotic described in Chapter 4.

One problem that does justify treatment is, however, mouth ulceration, though exactly what causes mouth ulceration is not properly understood. Remedies particular to such infection can be found in Chapter 1, page 16.

FUNGAL INFECTIONS OF THE MOUTH AND THROAT

Thrush and other throat and mouth fungal infections can be serious in themselves and provoke further infection elsewhere. The preparations used to treat them are, in most cases, the same as those used to treat such conditions elsewhere on the skin and genitalia. (*See* Chapter 6, page 83 for amphotericin and Chapters 4 and 6, pages 67–70 and 84, for miconazole and nystatin.) Precautions and reactions duplicate those when the preparations are used for other parts of the body. Metronidazole has other applications for inflammation of the sexual organs; polynoxylin and dequalinium preparations are particular to oral fungal infections. All these drugs are fairly powerful, and even those which are available OTC as well as by prescription should be administered under the supervision of a physician.

Preparations commonly used

Active principal	Proprietary preparation	Dosage
Amphotericin	**Fungilin**	Lozenges—1 four times daily Paste—apply 2–4 times daily
Dequalinium	▲ **Dequadin** ▲ **Labosept**	Lozenges—1 every three hours
Metronidazole	**Flagyl**	Tablets—200 mg thrice daily
Miconazole	▲ **Daktarin**	Oral gel—5–10 ml retained in mouth four times daily
Nystatin	**Nystan**	Suspension—1 ml four times daily
Polynoxylin	▲ **Anaflex**	Throat lozenges, six to ten times daily

OTC MOUTHWASHES FOR GENERAL ORAL HYGIENE

These three OTC proprietary preparations are probably the best-known and most widely-used of the many general preparations on the market. They are used both for 'killing germs' when a cold or sore throat is threatened or established, and for banishing 'bad breath'. The cautions expressed at the beginning of this chapter hold for these remedies: while useful in some short-term problems, reliance on them can cause as many problems as it solves.

Proprietary preparation	Components
▲ **Listerine Antiseptic**	Alcohol, benzoic acid, eucalyptol, menthol, methyl salicylate, thymol
▲ **Dettol Mouthwash**	Chloroxylenol
▲ **TCP Antiseptic**	Combined chlorine, iodine and phenol

OTHER PREPARATIONS USED IN THE MOUTH

Active principal	Proprietary preparation
Acetarsol	▲ **Pyorex**
Anthraquinone	▲ **Pyralvex**
Benzydamine	▲ **Difflam Oral Rinse**
Cetylpyridinium	▲ **Merocets**

Table continued on next page

Other preparations used in the mouth *continued*

Active principal	*Proprietary preparation*
Chlorhexidine	▲ Corsodyl
	▲ Eludril
Domiphen bromide	▲ Bradosol
Fusafungine	Locabiotal
Hexetidine	▲ Oraldene
Phenol	▲ Chloraseptic
Povidone-iodine	▲ Betadine Mouth Wash

General note: No special precautions are necessary, if use is occasional; excessive use (the sensible maximum is four usages daily for five days) can produce secondary symptoms or soreness and inflammation. Rare sensitivity reactions also occur.

● *Special advantages:* Chlorhexidine preparations inhibit plaque formation on the teeth and this may prevent dental decay.

Chapter

15

TREATING PROBLEMS OF THE NERVES

One of the most common uses of tranquillisers is for relieving anxiety. At the same time they can promote sleep if given in a large dose at night. In other words, the relationship between a so-called tranquilliser and a sleeping tablet may well be a matter of dosage. However, it is necessary to point out that drugs that are excreted slowly by the body (say over six or eight hours) work better as sleeping tablets than those that the body eliminates quickly. This has led to certain remedies being prescribed as sleeping pills and others as tranquillisers. Note that all drugs in this chapter are available only on prescription, except for promethazine (Phenergan).

Drugs that sedate, control anxiety and promote sleep

In the past the commonest sedatives used were drugs belonging to the *barbiturate* family. They were widely prescribed for many years and doctors and patients got to know their advantages and dangers very well. These drugs have always been potentially hazardous in cases of overdosage; taken in high doses they not only sedate the mind very efficiently (which is the therapeutic effect sought in the use of tranquillisers and sleeping pills) but they also sedate that part of the brain that controls breathing. In cases of barbiturate intoxication the patient stops breathing and, unless promptly respirated artificially, dies.

The new families of tranquillisers and sedatives have much better safety factors than the barbiturates. When these new drugs were being developed it was hoped that they would be an improvement over one particularly hazardous characteristic of the barbiturates—their known propensity to cause habituation and their association with the 'withdrawal' symptoms that occur on cessation of therapy. To some extent this high hope has not been substantiated. Modern research is busy building up evidence that most of the new 'safe' drugs in this field still have some inherent hazards. Listed below are some drugs that control anxiety (tranquillisers) and promote sleep (sedatives).

THE NON-BARBITURATE DRUGS

Drugs commonly used as tranquillisers (T)
[those with sleep-inducing qualities (S) are noted]
Many of these drugs have side effects which are similar to those produced by the active principal of diazepam. These are generally drowsiness, dizziness, unsteadiness and a 'dry' mouth. In rare cases, diazepam can cause allergy and in cases of high dosage, a depression of the breathing reflexes. The special advantage of diazepam is that it is normally well tolerated, and that the effects of this tranquilliser have been well documented and observed.

ALPAZOLAM (T)

Xanax

● *Basic precautions:* As for diazepam.
● *Proper dosage:* 0.25–1 mg daily.
● *Side effects:* As for diazepam, but probably less intense.
● *Special advantages:* May be effective in treatment of mixed anxiety/depression states.

BENZOCTAMINE (T)

Tacitin

● *Basic precautions:* Avoid alcohol and driving. Not suitable for patients with severe liver or kidney disease.
● *Proper dosage:* 10–20 mg tablets thrice daily.
● *Side effects:* Dry mouth common; oversedation; stomach upsets.
● *Special advantages:* Is a useful muscle relaxant.

BROMAZEPAM (T)

Lexotan

● *Basic precautions:* As for diazepam.
● *Proper dosage:* 3–6 mg twice daily or at night.
● *Side effects:* As for diazepam.

CHLORDIAZEPOXIDE (T)

Librium, Tropium and Chlordiazepoxide (F)

● *Basic precautions:* Avoid alcohol, driving and operation of machinery.
● *Proper dosage:* 10–100 mg daily. Usual range 10–30 mg in divided doses. Elderly or debilitated patients should start with 10 mg daily.
● *Side effects:* As for diazepam; unsteadiness and drowsiness most likely.
● *Special advantages:* There are only mild side effects.

CHLORMEZANONE (T + S)

Trancopal

● *Basic precautions:* Do not combine with monoamine inhibitors (MAOI) (*see* pages 164–165) or phenothiazines, used primarily in treatment of schizophrenia (*see* pages 168–169), or alcohol. Do not drive or operate machinery.
● *Proper dosage:* 200 mg thrice daily, 200–400 mg at night.
● *Side effects:* As for diazepam.
● *Special advantages:* Flushing, skin rashes, relaxes painful muscles.

CLOBAZAM (T)

Frisium

- *Basic precautions:* Avoid alcohol, driving, operating machinery. Small doses advisable for patients with kidney or liver disease.
- *Proper dosage:* 20–30 mg daily or as single night-time dose. Dosage should be low for elderly.
- *Side effects:* Mild diazepam-type effects.
- *Special advantages:* Once daily dosage improves patient compliance. There is some evidence to suggest that there is minimal risk in terms of driving and machinery operation. Can be safely combined with antidepression drugs.

CLORAZEPATE (T + S)

Tranxene

- *Basic precautions:* As for diazepam. May potentiate alcohol, barbiturates, phenothiazine (used in treatment of schizophrenia, *see* pages 168–169).
- *Proper dosage:* One 15 mg capsule at night; up to three 7.5 mg capsules daily as single or divided doses.
- *Side effects:* As for diazepam.
- *Special advantages:* Once daily dosage helps patient compliance. Minor side effects.

DIAZEPAM (T + S)

Atensine, Evacalm, Sedapam, Solis, Tensium, Valium, Valrelease and Diazepam (F)

- *Basic precautions:* To be taken with caution by patients with neuromuscular disease, closed-angle glaucoma, respiratory disease, liver or kidney disease; for the elderly dosages should be reduced. Do not mix with alcohol, exercise care in driving and machinery operation. Prolonged use may lead to dependency. Gradual withdrawal after long-term use.
- *Proper dosage:* 2–30 mg daily in divided doses or single dose at night.
- *Side effects:* Drowsiness, dizziness, unsteadiness, dry mouth, rare allergy, depression of breathing reflexes in high dosage. Breakdown of inhibitions, especially when alcohol consumed.
- *Special advantages:* On the whole well tolerated. Possibly the best documented drug to be used as a tranquilliser.

HYDROXYZINE (T)

Atarax

- *Basic precautions:* May potentiate other sedatives.
- *Proper dosage:* 25–100 mg four times daily; dosage adjusted to suit response.
- *Side effects:* Slight drowsiness and dryness of mouth.
- *Special advantages:* A rapid-action, highly selective tranquilliser, which relaxes muscles. It also has an antispasmodic, antisickness and antihistamine action. Enhances pain-killing effect of morphine-like drugs.

KETAZOLAM (T)

Anxon

- *Basic precautions:* May potentiate other sedatives, especially alcohol, antidepressive drugs, painkillers and anaesthetics. Care to be exercised if driving or operating machinery.

- *Proper dosage:* 15–60 mg daily.
- *Side effects:* Some drowsiness.
- *Special advantages:* Once daily dosage helps patient compliance; helps to reduce muscle spasticity associated with multiple sclerosis, or after strokes and injury.

LORAZEPAM (T + S)
Ativan
- *Basic precautions:* As for diazepam.
- *Proper dosage:* 10 mg daily in divided dosage or 4 mg at night.
- *Side effects:* As for diazepam. Habituation especially well-documented with regular use.
- *Special advantages:* As for diazepam; it may also help in treating phobias and obsessional states.

MEDAZEPAM (T + S)
Nobrium
- *Basic precautions:* As for diazepam.
- *Proper dosage:* 5 mg at one time, increasing up to four times daily until maximum effect is maintained.
- *Side effects:* As for diazepam, but less drowsiness.
- *Special advantages:* Claimed to sedate without interfering with powers of concentration.

MEPROBAMATE (T)
Equanil, Meprate, Milonorm, Miltown, Tenavoid
(also contains bendrofluazide) **and Meprobamate (F)**
- *Basic precautions:* Not suitable for patients with epilepsy or porphyria. May carry relatively high risk of dependency.
- *Proper dosage:* 400 mg at night. Unsuitable for daytime sedation.
- *Side effects:* Drowsiness and diazepam-type symptoms; other effects are gastro-intestinal disturbances, skin 'creepiness', weakness, headache, sometimes over-excitement, visual disturbances, blood abnormalities.
- *Special advantages:* None—rarely used today.

OXAZEPAM (T)
Serenid-D, Serenid Forte
- *Basic precautions:* As for diazepam.
- *Proper dosage:* 10–30 mg up to four times daily.
- *Side effects:* As for diazepam. Other side effects include vertigo, dizziness, headache, tremor, excitation, altered sex drive, rashes.
- *Special advantages:* Short-acting tranquilliser.

PROPRANOLOL (T)
Berkolol, Inderal, Inderal LA and Propranolol tablets (F)
- *Basic precautions:* Check drug interaction table. Not suitable for patients with asthma, heart failure, some artery diseases or in pregnancy. Should not be used after prolonged fasting or by diabetics.
- *Proper dosage:* In divided doses from 30–320 mg per day as directed by the physician. *Special note:* discontinuance of dose should be gradual, preferably over several days.

- *Side effects:* Common side effects include heart decompensation symptoms (breathlessness), oedema, cold extremities, exercise pain in legs, over-slowing of pulse, wheeziness, sometimes vivid dreams and hallucinations on high doses. Lassitude and 'dry-eyes' reported. Impotence a common adverse effect.
- *Special advantages:* Used for treating anxiety and controlling tremor. Also a well-tried *beta*-blocker much used for the control of blood pressure, angina and symptoms arising from an irregular heart action. These drugs are also used to remedy overaction of thyroid gland as are some other *beta*-blockers. (*See* section on thyroid remedies, Chapter 5.)

Non-barbiturates used to promote sleep (S)

CHLORAL HYDRATE
Noctec and Chloral mixture (F)
- *Basic precautions:* Not suitable for patients with severe liver, heart or kidney disease, gastritis or peptic ulcer. Special caution is needed if patient is on coumarin-type anticoagulants. Alcohol potentiates its effects. Habituation can occur. May enhance action of strong analgesics if excessive doses given.
- *Proper dosage:* 0.5–1 g at night, taken with water.
- *Side effects:* Gastritis; rarely a state of excitement.
- *Special advantages:* Rapid action—within 30 minutes.

CHLORMETHIAZOLE
Heminevrin
- *Basic precautions:* Not suitable for patients with severe liver disease. May potentiate alcohol or other sedatives. To be used with caution by the addiction-prone. May interfere with driving or operating machinery the day after drug has been taken.
- *Proper dosage:* 2 capsules at night.
- *Side effects:* Tingling in the nose, sneezing, eye-watering, headache, gastro-intestinal upset.
- *Special advantages:* The 'hangover' sensation is generally slight.

DICHLORALPHENAZONE
Welldorm
- *Basic precautions:* As for chloral hydrate.
- *Proper dosage:* 2–3 tablets with a drink, 20 minutes before bedtime.
- *Side effects:* As for chloral hydrate.
- *Special advantages:* As for chloral hydrate, but slightly less irritating to stomach.

FLURAZEPAM
Dalmane
- *Basic precautions:* Avoid alcohol.
- *Proper dosage:* 15–30 mg at night, half an hour before retiring.
- *Side effects:* Morning drowsiness, dizziness, unsteadiness. Bitter aftertaste.
- *Special advantages:* Useful for treating disturbed sleep with much night and early morning waking.

NITRAZEPAM
Mogadon, Nitrados, Remnos, Somnite, Surem and Nitrazepam (F)

- *Basic precautions:* These drugs may modify driving ability, operation of machinery next day. Avoid prolonged use. Do not exceed prescribed dosage or withdraw drug abruptly. Use with caution for patients with chest, liver and kidney disease. *See* drug interaction table. Individual response very variable; dosage must be carefully adjusted for each patient. Dependence potential equals that of diazepam.
- *Proper dosage:* 5–20 mg before retiring.
- *Side effects:* The 'hangover' effect is common; occasional confusion, dry mouth. Rare allergic reactions.
- *Special advantages:* A well tested and very safe night sedative. Over one hundred times the normal dose has been taken with impunity.

TEMAZEPAM
Normison, Euhypnos

- *Basic precautions:* As for nitrazepam.
- *Proper dosage:* 10–60 mg on retiring.
- *Side effects:* Minimal 'hangover' effect.
- *Special advantages:* Rapid action and few side effects.

PROMETHAZINE
▲ Phenergan and Promethazine (F)

- *Basic precautions:* Should be used with caution as some patients are hypersensitive to its action. Avoid alcohol.
- *Proper dosage:* 25–50 mg at night.
- *Side effects:* Rarely disorientation, also headache, twitching of limbs, nightmares and sun reaction. Cross-sensitivity to other major tranquillisers. Frequent or routine use, if not medically prescribed, is inadvisable.
- *Special advantages:* A good and safe sleeping tablet for occasional use.

General note: An earlier formulation, Persomnia, suggested a hypnotic/sedative action. Now it only contains analgesics, paracetamol and salicylamide. It is only an aid to sleep insofar as it may lessen pain which may be preventing sleep.

SEDATIVES BASED ON BARBITURATES AND OTHER SIMILAR DRUGS

Preparations commonly used

Active principal	Major use	Proprietary preparation	Formulary preparation	Dosage per day/night
Amylobarbitone	S	Amytal		60–200 mg
		Sodium Amytal		60–200 mg
		Tuinal		60–200 mg
			Amylobarbitone	60–200 mg
Butobarbitone	S	Soneryl		100 mg
			Butobarbitone	100 mg

Active principal	Major use	Proprietary preparation	Formulary preparation	Dosage per day/night
Cyclobarbitone	S	Evidorm Phanodorm		$\frac{1}{2}$–1 tablet 100–200 mg
			Cyclobarbitone	100–200 mg
Glutethimide	S	Doriden		250–500 mg
Heptabarbitone	S	Medomin		200–400 mg
Methyprylone	S	Noludar		200–400 mg
Pentobarbitone	S	Nembutal		100–200 mg
			Phenobarbitone	30 mg
Quinalbarbitone	S	Seconal		50–100 mg

- *Basic precautions:* Avoid use generally, since preparations can cause dependence, rebound insomnia and excessive sedation. Is not advised for patients suffering from porphyria, respiratory ailments or impaired liver function. Special caution is advised with reference to alcohol potentiation. Next-day 'hangover' effect may prevent operation of machinery and driving. Consult your doctor if you are on anticoagulants.
- *Proper dosage:* As indicated in table.
- *Side effects:* Drowsiness next day, depression, headache. Sometimes paradoxical excitement precedes sleep following high doses. Abrupt withdrawal can produce fits. Confusion and unsteadiness are common in the elderly. Accidental over-dosage common. General depression of the central nervous system.
- *Special advantages:* May have special medical uses when more modern drugs have become ineffective. Were widely prescribed until about ten years ago.

Treating psychosis and related illnesses

The term psychosis is to a large extent technical and arbitrary, and therefore really deserves explanation. A psychiatrist will usually keep the term psychosis to describe a mental illness which is severe, produces conspicuously disordered behaviour and cannot be understood as an exaggeration of an ordinary experience. The victim may, in some cases, be without insight into his condition. Examples of psychosis include schizophrenia, manic-depression—in these, changes in the brain cannot be identified with any clarity (if at all); there are other diseases in which altered brain anatomy (brain damage and so on) can be demonstrated.

Related to psychosis is a large group of mental illnesses called psychoneuroses. These are less serious, and the patient retains an insight into his condition. Personality change and deterioration does not occur and the patient is not confused. To a large extent, therefore, it is obvious that psychosis and psycho-neurosis (examples of which include anxiety reactions, phobias and general 'neurotic' ill-health) are very different types of illness. This is interesting because, from the point of view of treatment, there is some therapeutic overlap. There exist many cases of 'borderline' psychoses/neurosis, and these cases require careful adjustment of their drug regimen, sometimes combining sedating drugs (*see* pages 153–159) with one or more of the preparations below.

For ease of identification and practical application, remedies will be considered under two headings:
(i) Remedies commonly used to treat depression and mania;
(ii) Remedies commonly used in the management of schizophrenia.

REMEDIES COMMONLY USED TO TREAT DEPRESSION AND MANIA

It may seem strange that these illnesses, which can feature two extremes of behaviour, are grouped together. But sometimes the pattern of illness is an alternating one and 'manic' behaviour alternates with depression. When the term 'depression' is used this must not be interpreted to mean 'feeling depressed'. Mood swings in which one day we may feel on top of the world and yet a day or two later feel down in the dumps are part of everyday living. Real depression—like mania—is a disease with characteristic signs and symptoms that can be recognised by a physician.

'Tricyclic' and other antidepressants

One group of antidepressants have been named 'tricyclic' because of their chemical structure. Medicines in this group are generally used for treating moderate to severe episodes of depressive illness. They are slow to begin acting (two to three weeks) and improvement in sleep pattern may be the first indication that the drug is working. Doses vary with individual needs and close cooperation between doctor and patient is necessary. Blood tests can sometimes indicate what level of dosage is necessary. The doctor will always be alert to the lack of response that occurs in almost 50 per cent of cases so that alternative treatments can be kept in mind. Once the depression lifts, both patient and doctor need to be in close touch so that the right moment for *slow* reduction of treatment, without relapse, can be chosen.

Apart from the usual features of a successful drug regime, this group of medicines, and others which are chemically related, call for special consideration. Side effects are common, but tolerance to some of them develops and so patients are encouraged to persevere and 'soldier on' in the treatment of their depression. Elderly folk have to take care when starting treatment as most remedies also lower blood pressure or can cause fainting attacks. It has to be stressed that tricyclic drugs may cause irregular heart rhythm—not only in patients with heart disease—and therefore must be used with caution. They can also, upon occasion, *increase* depression, so relatives and friends should be aware of this and of the possible resultant hazard of accidental or deliberate overdosage.

Active principal	Major use	Other use	Proprietary preparation	Formulary preparation
Amitriptyline	D	A & E	Domical Elavil Lentizol Saroten Tryptizol	Amitriptyline
Butriptyline	D	A	Evadyne	
Clomipramine	D	P & O	Anafranil	

Active principal	Major use	Other use	Proprietary preparation	Formulary preparation
Desipramine	D		Pertofran	
Dothiepin	D	A	Prothiaden	
Doxepin	D	A	Sinequan	
Imipramine	D	E	Berkomine Tofranil	
Iprindole	D		Prondol	
Maprotiline	D	A	Ludiomil	
Mianserin	D	A	Bolvidon Norval	
Nomifensine	D	A	Merital	
Nortriptyline	D	E	Allegron Aventyl	
Protriptyline	D	W	Concordin	
Trazodone	D	A	Molipaxin	
Trimipramine	D	A	Surmontil	
Viloxazine	D		Vivalan	
Zimelidine	D		Zelmid	

Note: The key indicates which disorder the drug is used for. D = depression, A = anxiety, E = enuresis, P = phobia, O = obsessive state, W = withdrawal.

General note: Amitryptyline is discussed as being typical of all drugs in this section and will be considered in detail. Then brief mention of the other similar drugs will be noted to emphasise special differences.

AMITRIPTYLINE

Domical, Elavil, Lentizol, Saroten, Tryptizol and Amitriptyline (F)

- *Basic precautions:* Special caution to be used if patients have epilepsy—may lessen epileptic 'threshold' for fits. Some sedation usually occurs and may affect driving ability or operation of machinery. Alcohol is best avoided. Not suitable after recent heart attack, or if mania is suspected. Should be avoided in conditions of glaucoma, pregnancy, diabetes or if there is difficulty in passing urine or if there is suspected liver ailment or enlargement of the prostate.
- *Proper dosage:* 30–75 mg (less in the elderly) daily, in divided doses, or sometimes as a single dose at bedtime. Dosage gradually adjusted to maximum of 225 mg per day if necessary.
- *Side effects:* Dry mouth, blurred vision, constipation, difficulty in passing water, fainting, sweating, trembling, rashes, sexual problems, impotency, dizziness, hypertension.
- *Special advantages:* Well tried antidepressant with a sedative action.

BUTRIPTYLINE
Evadyne
- *Proper dosage:* 25 mg thrice daily, increased as necessary to 150 mg daily.
- *Special advantages:* Also reduces anxiety.

CLOMIPRAMINE
Anafranil
- *Proper dosage:* 25–100 mg daily in divided doses or as single bedtime dose. Increased to 150 mg daily if necessary or to 150 mg if used for treatment of phobias or obsessional states.
- *Special advantages:* Useful also for treating phobias or obsessional states.

DESIPRAMINE
Pertofran
- *Proper dosage:* 25 mg thrice daily. Increased as necessary to 50 mg four times daily.

DOTHIEPIN
Prothiaden
- *Proper dosage:* 75–150 mg daily in divided doses or as single bedtime dose.
- *Special advantages:* If insomnia is a particular feature of complaint, Prothiaden may be helpful; more sedative than amitriptyline.

DOXEPIN
Sinequan
- *Proper dosage:* 30–75 mg daily or at bedtime, increasing to 300 mg if necessary,
- *Special advantages:* Claimed to be less likely to cause side effects affecting the heart.

IMIPRAMINE
Berkomine, Tofranil
- *Proper dosage:* 75 mg daily in divided doses or at bedtime, increased to a maximum 225 mg if necessary.
- *Special advantages:* Less sedating than amitriptyline but greater tendency to create other side effects.

IPRINDOLE
Prondol
- *Proper dosage:* 15–30 mg thrice daily, increased to a maximum of 60 mg thrice daily if necessary.
- *Side effects:* Jaundice in rare cases.
- *Special advantages:* Few and mild side effects.

MAPROTILINE
Ludiomil
- *Proper dosage:* 25–150 mg daily in divided doses or single bedtime dose. Increased as necessary to 300 mg.
- *Special advantages:* Lowers convulsive threshold.

MIANSERIN
Bolvidon, Norval
- *Proper dosage:* 30–40 mg daily in divided doses or at bedtime; increased gradually to 200 mg if necessary.
- *Special advantages:* Few and mild side effects.

NOMIFENSINE
Merital
- *Proper dosage:* 20–50 mg two to three times daily, increased if necessary to 200 mg daily.
- *Special advantages:* Few and mild side effects. Onset of action may be shorter (eg 7–10 days versus 3–4 weeks) for this drug than for other drugs in the group.

NORTRIPTYLINE
Allegron, Aventyl
- *Proper dosage:* 10 mg two to four times daily, increased if necessary to 100 mg daily.
- *Special advantages:* Less sedating, but it causes more bladder problems, mouth dryness and blurred vision.

PROTRIPTYLINE
Concordin
- *Proper dosage:* 5–10 mg three to four times daily, not to be taken later than 4 pm. Increased if necessary to 60 mg daily.
- *Side effects:* More common side effects relating to the heart and fainting. May aggravate tension, anxiety, insomnia. Also photosensitisation and rashes reported (avoid direct sunlight). Use with special caution for the elderly.
- *Special advantages:* Useful if apathy and withdrawal become problems.

TRAZODONE
Molipaxin
- *General note:* Chemically unrelated to tricyclic antidepressants, this drug is similar in action to amitriptyline.
- *Basic precautions:* Although there are no absolute contra-indications, care should be taken in use by persons with liver and kidney damage.
- *Proper dosage:* 100–150 mg daily and then increased to 200–300 mg at end of first week. Rarely increased to 600 mg daily in divided doses. For the elderly not more than 100 mg doses. Gradual reduction when possible.
- *Side effects:* Sedation, more rarely dizziness, headache, gastrointestinal symptoms, dry mouth, tremor, constipation, blurred vision, restlessness.
- *Special advantages:* Rare side effects; also helps with anxiety.

TRIMIPRAMINE
Surmontil
- *Basic precautions:* Use with special caution for patients with liver disease.
- *Proper dosage:* 50–75 mg daily in divided doses or as single dose two hours before bedtime. Increased if necessary to 300 mg daily.
- *Side effects:* Dry mouth, fainting, prominent pins and needles.
- *Special advantages:* One of the most sedative of antidepressants.

VILOXAZINE
Vivalan
- *Basic precautions:* If antihypertensives or phenytoin are concurrently taken, dosage of these may need to be modified.

- *Proper dosage:* 50–100 mg two to three times daily; increased if necessary to 400 mg daily.
- *Side effects:* Headache and rashes, dyspepsia.
- *Special advantages:* Especially well tolerated by the elderly.

ZIMELIDINE
Zelmid

- *Basic precautions:* Not to be recommended if mania present.
- *Proper dosage:* 100–200 mg in morning as single dose.
- *Side effects:* As for amitriptyline. May enhance appetite.
- *Special advantages:* Less toxic than other tricyclics.

The MAOI antidepressants

The term MAOI is really an acronym for monoamine-oxidase inhibitor. It refers to the enzyme in the brain and the manner in which the drug affects it. The term was coined by the scientists who developed this kind of therapy and it has now entered popular parlance.

The MAOI antidepressants are very powerful drugs and they are generally used only for cases that have not already responded to other forms of treatment. These drugs can be the cause of considerable interaction problems with other drugs and they also react adversely, and possibly dangerously, with several foods. Therefore all patients should be in possession of a MAOI treatment card before they start therapy.

> **TREATMENT CARD**
> *Carry this card with you at all times. Show it to any doctor who may treat you other than the doctor who prescribed this medicine, and to your dentist if you require dental treatment.*
>
> **INSTRUCTIONS TO PATIENTS**
> **Please read carefully**
> While taking this medicine and for 10 days after your treatment finishes you must observe the following simple instructions:—
> 1 Do not eat CHEESE, PICKLED HERRING OR BROAD BEAN PODS.
> 2 Do not eat or drink BOVRIL, OXO, MARMITE or ANY SIMILAR MEAT OR YEAST EXTRACT.
> 3 Do not take any other MEDICINES (including tablets, capsules, nose drops, inhalations or suppositories) whether purchased by you or previously prescribed by your doctor, without first consulting your doctor or your pharmacist.
> NB *Treatment for coughs and colds, pain relievers and tonics are medicines.*
> 4 Drink ALCOHOL only in moderation and avoid CHIANTI WINE completely.
> **Report any severe symptoms to your doctor and follow any other advice given by him.**
>
> M.A.O.I.   Prepared by The Pharmaceutical Society and the British Medical Association on behalf of the Health Departments of the United Kingdom.

PHENELZINE
Nardil

- *Basic precautions:* Read treatment card. Not to be taken within two weeks of taking tricyclic antidepressants; should not be taken by persons with coeliac disease, gluten enteropathy, cerebrovascular disease, liver damage. Not suitable for use within two weeks of surgery or dentistry. Great care needed for elderly or agitated patients and those with blood diseases or diabetes.

- *Proper dosage:* 15 mg thrice daily. If no response is apparent in one week, then four times daily. Once response obtained, gradual reduction of dosage may occur.
- *Side effects:* Dizziness, drowsiness, fatigue, leg swelling, intestinal upset, insomnia, blurred vision. Less commonly—headache, nervousness, pins and needles, increased appetite, rashes, difficulty in passing urine, tremor, excitement.
- *Special advantages:* Useful for treating depression, especially with phobic symptoms.

IPRONIAZID
Marsilid

- *Basic precautions:* Special care necessary in cases of kidney disease. *See* drug interaction table; read treatment card. Avoid alcohol, driving, operation of machinery.
- *Proper dosage:* 100–150 mg daily until improvement allows reduction to 25 or 50 mg daily.
- *Side effects:* Constipation, difficulty in passing urine, dizziness, insomnia, impotence, tremor, unsteadiness, jaundice, headache. (This last is often an early sign of drug interaction or overdosage). May cause fits in epileptics. Other antidepressants should be withheld until 14 days after Marsilid therapy has ended. Tends to have a cumulative and persistent action.

TRANYLCYPROMINE
Parnate

- *Basic precautions:* Not to be taken until at least two weeks, preferably four, have passed after the use of other antidepressants; allow one week to elapse after taking Parnate before starting with any other medicine with which it may react. Read treatment card. Not suitable for patients of cerebrovascular, heart, liver and blood diseases. Special care needed in use by the elderly and epileptics.
- *Proper dosage:* 10–40 mg daily. If no response is evident in one week, add a further midday tablet. After response is achieved, reduce to 10 mg daily.
- *Side effects:* Insomnia, dizziness, muscle weakness, dry mouth. Throbbing headache indicates high blood pressure—treatment should be withdrawn immediately.
- *Special advantages:* Not so toxic to liver as some other MAOIs.

Other antidepressants
This group includes some mixed remedies that are, generally speaking, not much prescribed because the individual components rarely match the patient's needs. It also includes other compounds found useful in certain types of depression.

Active principal	Major use	Other use	Proprietary preparation
Flupenthixol	D	A & W	**Fluanxol**
Tofenacin	D		**Elamol**
Trazodone	D	A	**Molipaxin**
Tryptophan	D	M	**Optimax**
	D	M	**Optimax WV**
	D	M	**Pacitron**

Key: D = depression; A = anxiety; W = withdrawal; M = mania.

FLUPENTHIXOL
Fluanxol

- *Basic precautions:* To be used with special care for patients with Parkinson's disease, arteriosclerosis, heart disease, senile confusion or with excitable or overactive patients.
- *Proper dosage:* 1 mg in the morning and again before 4 pm in afternoon. Increase each dose by 0.5 mg to 3 mg daily if necessary. Reduce to 0.5 mg, to be taken twice daily, as possible.
- *Side effects:* Restlessness alternating with sedation. Occasionally insomnia.
- *Special advantages:* Effective in depression complicated by fatigue, apathy, or despondency. Also when poor initiative is a feature or obsessive tendencies are present. Apparently no habituation problems.

TOFENACIN
Elamol

- *Basic precautions:* Not suitable for patients with glaucoma, prostate disease, or when suicidal tendency is present.
- *Proper dosage:* 80–240 mg daily in divided doses.
- *Side effects:* Dry mouth, visual disturbance, tremor; rarely gastrointestinal upset, drowsiness, vertigo, agitation, rashes.
- *Special advantages:* Useful in mild to moderate depression in the elderly.

TRYPTOPHAN
Optimax, Optimax WV, Pacitron

- *Basic precautions:* Should not be prescribed for patients with bladder disease or Parkinson's disease. If used with MAOI it may potentiate their effect.
- *Proper dosage:* 1 g thrice daily, increasing to 6 g daily if necessary. Minimum treatment of four weeks is necessary.
- *Side effects:* Nausea, drowsiness.
- *Special advantages:* A safe antidepressant that can be combined with other drugs.

Remedies for treating isolated mania

Mania is a medical term used to describe a condition that may alternate with depression, but which may occur as an isolated disease. Mania may be characterised by overactivity and excessive restlessness or by extravagant and unusual behaviour—for instance in an attack of mania a man may decide to hire a plane to go on holiday or make social arrangements for entirely inappropriate entertainment of friends and colleagues. Treatment of manic symptoms may merely demand the prescription of sedatives, but in more worrying cases medicines containing lithium are often prescribed. These work very well in some, but certainly not all, cases, but have a narrow margin of safety. In other words, the dose necessary to provide a therapeutic effect is near to that which may be dangerous or even lethal. This being so, patients are carefully selected, usually by a psychiatrist, and are given lithium preparations while their blood is carefully monitored, so that therapeutic levels are both safe and adequate. Sometimes long-term treatment is necessary to prevent relapses of manic-depressive psychosis.

LITHIUM CARBONATE
Camcolit 250 and 400, Liskonum, Phasal, Priadel

- *Basic precautions:* Not suitable for patients with severe kidney or heart disease, Addison's disease or myxoedema. Dose adjustment is necessary if diarrhoea, vomiting or heavy sweating occurs. Caution in use for the elderly and patients on diuretics. Numerous drug interactions—acquaint your physician with other medications being used.
- *Proper dosage:* The drug regime must be closely supervised by doctor. 400–1200 mg are usually taken daily (in a single or divided dose). After four to five days a blood test should be taken to check levels and dose adjusted accordingly, indeed, regular blood tests should be given throughout treatment.
- *Side effects:* Mild gastrointestinal symptoms, dizziness, 'dazed' feeling, skin reactions. If any tendency to pass urine frequently develops, doctor should be informed. The same applies to increasing loss of appetite, gastrointestinal symptoms (diarrhoea, vomiting), lack of coordination, muscle weakness, drowsiness, lethargy, ringing in ears, blurred vision, joint pains and muscle twitching as these symptoms may indicate severe, and possibly dangerous, toxicity.
- *Special advantages:* There are few effective remedies for mania—lithium helps in many cases. It can be used to prevent episodes of depression from reoccurring, although it can intensify some cases of depression.

REMEDIES COMMONLY USED IN THE MANAGEMENT OF SCHIZOPHRENIA

Most of these drugs tranquillise and do not produce paradoxical excitement. Although used mostly in schizophrenia, they have other uses in psychiatry. In schizophrenia they relieve the more florid manifestations of the disease, especially thought disorders and delusions. They also effectively control hallucinations. In many cases treatment has to be accepted on a long-term basis before it is effective, and many of these drugs are given by injection. Withdrawal has to be carefully managed if worrying relapses are to be avoided. Remedies are grouped with reference to their side effects.

It is as well to remember that schizophrenia is a term used to describe a group of illnesses whose basic causation is unknown. It has characteristic mental symptoms leading to a fragmentation of personality, thus its name. Though the victim undergoes experiences which are unfamiliar to him, nevertheless they are mostly exaggerations or extensions of familiar sensations. As a result of the fragmented personality misreading his sensations, thought processes, the emotions, drive and mobility may be disordered. The impression given to the observer is one of oddity. Understandably, remedies for such a complex state are not always very effective.

It is also pertinent to note that in the management of severe and disabling psychotic illnesses, drugs have to be prescribed that do have considerable side effects. The physician prescribing treatment in such cases has to decide to what extent the severity of the disease demands the acceptance of undesirable side effects. In some cases, it is possible to prevent the worst of these effects by prescription of yet another drug. But such cases require a high degree of diligence on the part of the prescribing physician.

GROUP 1—CHLORPROMAZINE, PROMAZINE
These drugs have pronounced sedative effects and moderate 'anticholinergic' (*see* pages 22–23) effects (dry mouth, constipation, difficulty in passing urine, blurred vision). They also lead to moderate 'extrapyramidal' effects such as abnormal face and body movements and Parkinson's-disease type symptoms.

GROUP 2—PERICYAZINE, THIORIDAZINE
They have moderate sedative effects, marked 'anticholinergic', and minimal extrapyramidal effects.

GROUP 3—FLUPHENAZINE, PERPHENAZINE, THIOPROPAZATE, TRIFLUOPERAZINE
With minimal sedative and 'anticholinergic' effects, but marked extrapyramidal side effects.

GROUP 4—INCLUDES BENPERIDOL, CHLORPROTHIXENE, CLOPENTHIXOL, DROPERIDOL, FLUPENTHIXOL, HALOPERIDOL, OXYPERTINE, PIMOZIDE
These tend to resemble Group 3 but are of different chemical derivative from Groups 1–3.

Preparations commonly used

Active principal	Proprietary preparation	Formulary preparation	Dosage
GROUP 1			
Chlorpromazine	**Chloractil** **Largactil**		
		Chlorpromazine	20 mg–1 g per day
Promazine	**Sparine**		25–100 mg three to four times daily
GROUP 2			
Pericyazine	**Neulactil**		15–30 mg in two doses
Thioridazine	**Melleril**		150–600 mg per day
GROUP 3			
Fluphenazine	**Moditen**		2.5–10 mg per day in single dose
Perphenazine	**Fentazin**		4–24 mg daily in divided doses
Thiopropazate	**Dartalan**		10 mg thrice daily
Trifluoperazine	**Stelazine**		5 mg twice daily
GROUP 4			
Benperidol	**Anquil**		0.25–1.5 mg per day in divided doses
Chlorprothixene	**Taractan**		30–400 mg per day
Clopenthixol	**Clopixol**		20–200 mg daily in divided doses
Droperidol	**Droleptan**		5–20 mg per day
Flupenthixol	**Depixol**		3–18 mg per day
Haloperidol	**Haldol** **Serenace**		
		Haloperidol	0.5–5 mg two to three times daily
Oxypertine	**Integrin**		80–120 mg per day
Pimozide	**Orap**		2–20 mg per day

GROUP 1
- *Basic precautions:* To be used with care for patients with heart and blood vessel disease, Parkinson's disease, kidney or liver disease or a past history of jaundice. Avoid alcohol. Reduced dosage is necessary for the elderly.
- *Proper dosage: See* chart.
- *Side effects:* Some sedation may occur to start with, so care in driving and use of machinery is necessary.
- *Special advantages:* Have marked psychocorrective features.

GROUP 2
- *Basic precautions:* As for Group 1 drugs.
- *Proper dosage: See* chart.
- *Side effects:* Neulactil (*see* note above on Group 2 drugs). As for Group 1 drugs, except Melleril, which may produce brownish colouring of vision and male sexual dysfunction.
- *Special advantages:* Neulactil inhibits aggression and impulsiveness. Melleril has few side effects and is well tolerated.

GROUP 3
- *Basic precautions and side effects:* As for Group 1 drugs.
- *Proper dosage: See* chart.
- *Special advantages:* These remedies have tranquillising, antiagitation and anti-hostility effects. They also have an antiemetic (antisickness) effect.

GROUP 4
- *Basic precautions and side effects:* As for Group 1 drugs. Integrin not to be given within three weeks of MAOI drugs.
- *Proper dosage: See* chart.
- *Special advantages:* Anquil—used for deviant and antisocial sexual behaviour. Haldol and Serenace—broad-spectrum antipsychotic drugs which are also used to treat alcohol withdrawal symptoms and tics, stuttering and hiccough. Droleptan—used for rapid calming of manic or agitated patients. Taractan—a wide-spectrum antipsychotic. It is sedating but does not aggravate depression. Orap—controls hallucinations and thought disorders. In low dose it is beneficial in overactivity and aggression. Depixol—has alerting and antianxiety effect in higher doses. Integrin—antipsychotic and antimania properties.

Long-acting, single-injection (depot) drugs
For maintenance therapy these are often used. They are outside the general scope of this book.

The control of epilepsy

Epilepsy is a disease that can manifest itself at almost any age and close cooperation between the patient, the doctor and perhaps a patients' association—like the British Epilepsy Association—all helps to keep the illness controlled. The corner-stone of all treatment is adequate long-term medication, a point often overlooked by epileptics and their families. This is because of the 'knock-on' effect of anticonvulsant drug action. Such is the nature of epilepsy that, to some extent at least, 'fits breed fits'. 'Risking a fit', by reducing or stopping treatment, may not risk just *one* fit, but a whole group of seizures.

Another point not always appreciated by everybody is the very variable nature of this puzzling illness. One patient's epilepsy might mean one fit in a lifetime—another may suffer very frequent and disrupting seizures. Drug treatment, therefore, must be tailored to match all situations as far as possible—a fairly difficult state of affairs.

From the medical point of view, the control of epilepsy is simple, although far from fully effective, it is to suppress fits by maintaining enough of the anticonvulsant drug in the body at all times. The dose and frequency of medication is determined by the 'half life' of the drug and careful adjustment of doses until fits are controlled. Overdose effects may limit use of the remedy and indicate a change of treatment. The concept of half life is based on the time that half of the drug is still active within the body. It is also an index of the rate of breakdown of a drug by the body and a guide to its elimination. Monitoring dosage through blood analysis is often advisable. Some drugs like phenobarbitone have a long half life: they should be given just once a day. Others have a short half life measured only in hours.

The aim of all treatment is to control fits as simply and effectively as possible by as few tablets taken as infrequently as possible. The more complicated the routine, the more likelihood there is of the patient's failure to take medicines and the possibility of drug interaction. Once a regime that stops fits is arrived at it must be maintained until two years have passed without fits. Once it has been decided to reduce drug dosage, this must be done slowly if it is to be managed without drug-reduction fits being precipitated. The same care and overlap of therapy must be exercised when one type of drug is substituted for another.

Driving and epilepsy is an important subject. Patients may be allowed a driving licence if they have had a fit-free period of three years or there is evidence that fits have occurred only when sleeping at night. Some of the antiepileptic drugs in common use bear the warning (so prevalent in this book) that they may impair driving ability or make the operation of machinery generally unwise.

The relationship of epilepsy to drugs and pregnancy and dosage for children are subjects that are not dealt with generally in this book. Both pregnancy and the treatment of children are too intimate a subject to be dealt with generally, and must be a matter for consultation with a physician. One must stress however that, although many drugs used in the safe management of epilepsy can affect the foetus, in fact such effects are very rare. Quite often the risks of abrupt termination of treatment (because of production of seizures) is far more risky than the continuance during pregnancy of medication on medical advice.

THE THREE TYPES OF EPILEPTIC ATTACK

To set the complex subject of seizure control into perspective for patients and their families, aspects of medication will be examined by dividing them into groups that control various symptoms. Epilepsy, to some extent, seems tailored to its victims. In other words, the manifestation of the disease tends to 'run to form'—some patients suffering (mostly) *grand mal* attacks, others *petit mal* or *myoclonic jerks*. The term *most* is an important qualification, for some epileptics unfortunately experience mixed seizures.

Our general principle is to assume that all drugs are potentially hazardous in pregnancy until a physician decrees that the safety margin permits further treatment. Nonetheless, the epileptic woman who becomes pregnant or the pregnant woman who develops fits is a very special case: she must consult her doctor immediately, in the meanwhile continuing with any anticonvulsant drugs.

Drugs used for grand mal and focal epilepsy
General note: Some duplicated remedies have dual actions

CARBAMAZEPINE
Tegretol
● *Basic precautions:* Special care to be taken when patients have certain heart disease. Concurrent medication may need to be modified, especially when the contraceptive pill is being taken or anticoagulant therapy. Not to be taken with MAOIs or within two weeks of stopping MAOI drugs.
● *Proper dosage:* Dosage according to manufacturer's instructions, but has to be monitored. The usual is 100–200 mg a day—then adjusted according to response to a maximum 800 mg daily.
● *Side effects:* Dizziness, double vision, drowsiness, dry mouth, gastrointestinal upset, a generalised rash (3 per cent of takers). Rare cases of anaemia, jaundice, oedema.
● *Special advantages:* Effective therapy (also used in trigeminal neuralgia). May help in temporal lobe epilepsy.

CLONAZEPAM
Rivotril
● *Basic precautions:* Alcohol is forbidden, extra care if drug is part of multi-therapy regime.
● *Proper dosage:* Low dosages initially (1 mg daily), increasing to 8 mg daily in divided doses.
● *Side effects:* Fatigue, aggressiveness, irritability.
● *Special advantages:* Few side effects and minor toxicity.

ETHOTOIN
Peganone
● *Basic precautions:* None, but blood counts and urine tests should be carried out at monthly intervals. Other anticonvulsive treatment should not be discontinued abruptly.
● *Proper dosage:* 1–3 g daily in four to six divided doses, taken after food.
● *Side effects:* Occasionally occur as gastrointestinal upset, fatigue, dizziness, headache, double vision, rashes, numbness, fever and chest pain.
● *Special advantages:* Minimal incidence of side effects.

METHYLPHENOBARTITONE
Prominal
● *Basic precautions, etc:* Same as for phenobarbitone preparations below.

PHENOBARBITONE
Luminal, Parabal, Phenobarbitone Spansule and Phenobarbitone (F)
● *Basic precautions:* Not suitable for patients with porphyria, special care in use for elderly. Avoid mixing with alcohol and abrupt withdrawal.

- *Proper dosage:* 90–600 mg per day.
- *Side effects:* Drowsiness, lethargy, difficulty walking, rashes, occasionally excitement or confusion.
- *Special advantages:* Safe drugs if used carefully, bearing in mind dependence problems and cumulative action.

PHENYTOIN
Epanutin and Phenytoin (F)
- *Basic precautions:* Change over from other drugs should be made slowly and sudden withdrawal avoided. Caution should be exercised if there is a history of liver disease.
- *Proper dosage:* Best administered under blood-testing control. (Certain drugs may elevate blood levels of phenytoin.)
- *Side effects:* Gastrointestinal upset, nervousness, insomnia, unsteadiness, rare allergic reactions. Rarely gum and hair overgrowth.
- *Special advantages:* Provided drug is carefully monitored and right dosage stabilised, then Epanutin is an excellent anticonvulsant.

PRIMIDONE
Mysoline
- *Basic precautions:* None.
- *Proper dosage:* Treatment is started slowly with small doses (125 mg) taken late in the evening. Every third day dose is increased by 125 mg until 500 mg per day is taken. Then increased by 250 mg until attacks are controlled. Maximum dosage is 1.5 g. Total dose is best divided; if the attacks occur at night only or are associated with special circumstances (eg menstruation), dose may be modified.
- *Side effects:* Drowsiness, nausea, difficulty walking, visual disturbances and rashes, usually in very early stages of treatment—these may disappear on further treatment. Rarely, severe emotional upset occurs, also impotence, leg swelling and anaemia.
- *Special advantages:* Very effective anticonvulsant with generally low toxicity.

SODIUM VALPROATE
Epilim
- *Basic precautions:* Not suitable for patients with liver disease. Liver function tests should be carried out before treatment and at two-monthly intervals for six months. Blood tests are necessary before surgery. May produce false urine test results in diabetes.
- *Proper dosage:* 200 mg thrice daily after food, increasing by 200 mg per day at three-day intervals to a maximum of 2.6 g daily taken in divided doses.
- *Side effects:* Gastric upset, transient hair loss, swelling of legs, liver disease.
- *Special advantages:* Many; it is the *most* effective prophylactic antiepileptic agent available for most types of epilepsy.

SULTHIAME
Ospolot
- *Basic precautions:* Special care to be taken for patients with kidney disease. Changeover from other drugs should be carried out carefully over several weeks.
- *Proper dosage:* 100 mg twice daily raised to maximum of 200 mg thrice daily if necessary.

● *Side effects:* Mild side effects which subside in two weeks of treatment. They include an unusual feeling in face, gastric upset, giddiness, unsteadiness, breathlessness, loss of appetite.

● *Special advantages:* Mild and transient side effects.

Drugs used for petit mal

These are sometimes called absence seizures. Children are especially prone to this problem which, in some cases resembles a sudden loss of awareness or daydream state. In keeping with our general principle, no special doses are suggested for children. These must be a matter for medical advice and relative to child's age and weight.

CLONAZEPAM
Rivotril
For details: See page 171.

ETHOSUXIMIDE
Emeside, Zarontin and Ethosuximide (F)

● *Basic precautions:* Special care needed for patients of kidney or liver disease.

● *Proper dosage:* 500 mg increased by 250 mg every four to seven days until control is achieved. Maximum dosage 4 g.

● *Side effects:* Usually transient; they include apathy, drowsiness, depression, excitement, headache, unsteadiness, gastrointestinal upset, rashes, anaemia.

● *Special advantages:* Generally effective against petit mal.

SODIUM VALPROATE
Epilim
For details: See opposite page.

TROXIDONE
Tridione

● *Basic precautions:* Not suitable for patients with severe kidney, liver or blood diseases. Also not advised for persons with diseases of retina or optic nerve. Be ready to stop treatment promptly if rash or jaundice develop. Exacerbation of acne is a danger sign. Monthly blood counts and urine tests are necessary.

● *Proper dosage:* 0.9 g daily in divided dosage increased at one- or two-week intervals by 300 mg daily. Maximum dosage 1.8 g.

● *Side effects:* Sedation, 'glare' phenomenon (sensitivity to bright light), rashes, loss of appetite, bleeding of the nose, gums and vagina.

● *Special advantages:* Although quite toxic, a potent drug for petit mal.

Drugs for myoclonic (muscle) jerks

CLONAZEPAM
Rivotril
For details: See page 171.

SODIUM VALPROATE
Epilim
For details: See opposite page.

COMPOUND PREPARATIONS AND EPILEPSY

As with all compound preparations, the prescribing doctor has to battle against two opposing principles. Patients understandably do not like swallowing masses of different tablets and often tend to 'forget' to take those that seem to upset them—or do not help them. In other words, *compliance* is poor. On the other hand, convenient compound preparations are not always formulated to suit individual patient's needs. If tablet x contains twice as much of compound A than it does of compound B, and the patient really needs equal doses of A and B, then he is taking an improper dose. The three compound preparations, noted below, are in common use in epilepsy and suit many patients. Their side effects and other details can be assumed to be the result of a fair mix of their components (*see* pages 171–172).

Epanutin and Phenobarbitone capsules
Garoin (also contains phenytoin and phenobarbitone)
Mysoline and Phenytoin tablets

Treating Parkinson's disease

Parkinson's disease is an illness in which the brain fails to produce sufficient dopamine—a substance necessary to balance the nervous activity at certain functional areas in the brain. Therapy is aimed at adding dopamine-like substances to the circulation, and by giving drugs that tend to prevent dopamine breakdown. It is also possible to stimulate the receptor cells where dopamine actually works.

Another approach to therapy is to give drugs that control the worst symptoms of Parkinson's disease. This also has relevance to treatment of the allied condition, *Parkinsonism*. Parkinsonism can occur after a bout of encephalitis or may be secondary to another condition. Reactions to specific treatments in both Parkinson's disease and Parkinsonism is very variable. Often Parkinson's disease is first treated with symptom-controlling drugs and later with dopamine-like compounds, or symptom-controlling drugs are combined with other nerve-regulating drugs when levodopa cannot be prescribed.

Patients with either Parkinson's disease or Parkinsonism should consult the Parkinson's Disease Society, 36 Portland Place, London W1N 3DG (01-323 1174), for specialist guidance to management of their condition.

Dopamine-type drugs used in Parkinson's disease and Parkinsonism

AMANTADINE
Symmetrel
- *Basic precautions:* Not suitable for epileptics or for persons with peptic ulcer or severe kidney disease. May aggravate side effects of other anti-Parkinson's disease drugs. Use with caution for the confused or hallucinated. Concurrent use of nervous stimulants—ie certain slimming pills—can be dangerous.
- *Proper dosage:* 100 mg daily increased to twice daily; not to be taken later than early evening.
- *Side effects:* Rarely nervousness, dizziness, convulsing, hallucinations and rashes.
- *Special advantages:* A well tolerated drug.

BROMOCRIPTINE
Parlodel
- *Basic precautions:* Not suitable for people suffering from psychosis or severe heart/ blood vessel disease. It is a drug requiring very careful monitoring.
- *Proper dosage:* Always to be taken during a meal. Initially 1.25 mg at bedtime increasing after three days to 2.5 mg, then increased by 1.25 or 2.5 mg at three-day intervals until 30–40 mg daily is reached. Thereafter increased by 10 mg every three days until optimum dose (40–100 mg per day) is reached. In patients already on levodopa, dosage of this drug may be reduced as Parlodel is increased.
- *Side effects:* Nausea, dizziness, headache, vomiting, constipation.
- *Special advantages:* A valuable drug. Useful when levodopa has ceased to be effective.

LEVODOPA
Berkdopa, Brocadopa, Larodopa and Levodopa (F)
- *Basic precautions:* Not suitable for patients with narrow-angle glaucoma, severe psychoneurosis or psychosis; not to be used in conjunction with MAOI drugs or within two weeks of these; not to be taken by patients with malignant melanoma; and not to be taken concurrently with Vitamin B6 (which is found in many multivitamin tablets). Special care to be exercised when taken by persons with chest, heart, kidney and liver disease or when asthma or blood pressure treatment is necessary. Special care to be exercised during surgery.
- *Proper dosage:* 125 mg twice daily, taken immediately after food, increased after one week to 125 mg four to five times daily. Thereafter increased at weekly intervals by 375 mg daily. Normal range 2.5–8 g per day. Dose may be adjusted to give 'smooth' effect by two-hourly administration (62.5, 125 and 250 mg capsules available).
- *Side effects:* Side effects may develop after a period of tolerated dosage and fade with dose reduction. They include loss of appetite, gastrointestinal upset, dizziness, palpitation, excessive passing of urine and incontinence, discolouration of urine, abnormal involuntary movements and psychiatric symptoms.
- *Special advantages:* Gives worthwhile sustained relief in most patients. May take six months before maximum improvement occurs.

Madopar (also contains benserazide)
- *Basic precautions:* As for levodopa.
- *Proper dosage:* 1 capsule twice daily increased by 1 capsule every three days until effective dose (2–6 capsules) is maintained.
- *Side effects:* Less gastrointestinal side effects than 'plain' levodopa.
- *Special advantages:* More rapid response (one to three weeks). Less side effects.

Sinemet (also contains carbidopa)
- *Basic precautions:* As for levodopa.
- *Proper dosage:* Start with $\frac{1}{2}$ tablet once or twice daily, increased by $\frac{1}{2}$ tablet every other day until optimum dosage (3–6 tablets) is attained.
- *Special advantages:* Very rapid improvement. The carbidopa in Sinemet prevents breakdown of levodopa in the body and makes more available to the brain.

Symptom-correcting drugs for Parkinsonism

Active principal	Proprietary preparation	Formulary preparation	Dosage
Benzhexol	Artane	Benzhexol	1–2 mg increased to 5–15 mg in divided daily doses
Benztropine	Cogentin		500 micrograms increasing to 1–4 mg per day
Biperiden	Akineton		1 mg twice daily increasing to 2–6 mg daily
Methixene	Tremonil		2.5 mg thrice daily increasing to 15–60 mg daily
Orphenadrine	Disipal Norflex		150 mg increasing to 400 mg per day
Procyclidine	Kemadrin		2.5 mg thrice daily increasing to 60 mg daily

- *Basic precautions:* The drugs used to treat Parkinsonism generally have similar attributes. Therefore the basic precautions are also similar: care to be taken when prescribed for persons with urinary trouble, heart and kidney disease. Avoid abrupt termination of treatment. Not suitable for persons with glaucoma, or with certain slow-movement problems (tardive dyskinesia).
- *Special considerations:* Disipal—may cause insomnia, produce euphoria, and is more likely to control tremor. Cogentin—may sedate, so care to be taken when driving or operating machinery, avoid alcohol. Tremonil—more effective in tremor control than rigidity. Kemadrin—may cause drowsiness
- *Side effects:* Dry mouth, gastrointestinal upset, dizziness, blurred vision, nervousness, confusion, excitement, psychiatric disturbance.
- *Special advantages:* These drugs all work basically in the same way to counteract the worst symptoms of Parkinsonism. They produce about a 20 per cent reduction in tremor and rigidity in some patients. They help reduce excessive saliva production. They are particularly useful in treating Parkinsonism rather than Parkinson's disease.

Drugs used for choreas, tics and related disorders

In many diseases involuntary movements (sometimes referred to as tics or choreas) need treatment. Sometimes general sedatives will help, but more specific drugs are available and prescribed. They include haloperidol (*see* schizophrenia, pages 167–169) and tetrabenazine.

TETRABENAZINE
Nitoman

- *Basic precautions:* Special care needed if patient is taking levodopa.
- *Proper dosage:* 25 mg thrice daily increased by 25 mg per day every three or four days to a maximum, if tolerated, of 200 mg per day. If no improvement occurs in seven days it is unlikely to be a useful drug.
- *Side effects:* Drowsiness, dizziness, depression.
- *Special advantages:* Useful in illnesses where movement disorders predominate.

Chapter

16

REMEDIES THAT CONTROL PAIN

A philosopher remarked that 'pain and pleasure are simple ideas incapable of definition'. Pain is a personal experience of unpleasant sensations; it can be very variable and is modified by many factors including cultural, environmental, medical and psychological ones. Pain is sometimes a useful warning, but often a purposeless burden. As life expectancy increases, more of us become prey to degenerative diseases. Chronic pain, of one sort or another, becomes more commonplace.

Modern principles of pain control are humane: they stress that the withholding of good pain relief when it is needed, or prescribing by the clock rather than by the patient's needs is both unkind and inefficient. Quite often an over-zealous restriction of pain-relieving remedies is due to a mistaken fear of narcotic addiction. Pain, particularly severe pain, is psychologically destructive, a fact well appreciated by the torturer the world over. To ask a sick person also to bear the unnecessary burden of pain is inhumane patient management.

Painkillers are also called analgesics. Many analgesics have other properties; for instance they may be anti-inflammatory or antirheumatic (*see* Chapter 11).

Some painful conditions respond poorly to general painkillers. In these conditions drugs leave the stomach before they are dissolved and absorbed: they are less likely to cause irritation of the stomach lining. Claradin, Paynocil, Solprin/Disprin are soluble products; Laboprin also contains lysine.

General pain control

MILD TO MODERATE PAIN TREATMENT

Such a description of pain can vary greatly from person to person. But the general accepted definition would run to such problems as tension headache, muscle ache, toothache, sprain pain and backache.

Drugs commonly used

Active principal	Proprietary preparation	Formulary preparation
Aspirin	▲ Alka-Seltzer	
	▲ Aspergum	▲ Aspirin
	▲ Aspro and Aspro Clear	
	▲ Breoprin	▲ Aspirin Dispersible
	▲ Caprin	
	▲ Claradin	
	▲ Fynnon Calcium Asprin	
	▲ Genasprin	
	▲ Laboprin	
	▲ Levius	
	▲ Nu-Seals Aspirin	
	▲ Paynocil	
	▲ Solprin/Disprin	
Benorylate	▲ Benoral	
	▲ Triadol	
Codeine		Codeine Phosphate tablets and syrup
Dextropropoxyphene	Doloxene	
Dextropropoxyphene/paracetamol	Distalgesic	
Diflunisal	Dolobid	
Dihydrocodeine	DF 118	
Fenoprofen	Fenopron	
	Progesic	
Flufenamic acid	Meralen	
Mefenamic acid	Ponstan	
Naproxen	Synflex	
Paracetamol	▲ Calpol	▲ Paracetamol tablets and elixir
	▲ Hedex	
	▲ Panadol	
	▲ Panasorb	
	▲ Panets	
	▲ Salzone	
Pentazocine	Fortral	
Salsalate	Disalcid	
Sodium salicylate		▲ Sodium salicylate mixture

ASPIRIN

▲ (See table for proprietary and formulary preparations)

- *Basic precautions:* Not advisable for patients suffering from peptic ulceration, cerebral haemorrhage, haemophilia, those taking anticoagulants or antigout remedies (uricosurics) or those hypersensitive to aspirin.
- *Proper dosage:* 300–900 mg taken four-hourly after or with meals. Maximum dosage of 4 g per day.

- *Side effects:* Stomach pains, occasionally vomiting, wheeziness, gastric bleeding, skin rashes, ringing in ears.
- *Special advantages of proprietary preparations:* Aspergum is a chewing gum preparation; Breoprin, Caprin, Levius, Nu-Seals Aspirin are enteric-coated preparations which leave the stomach before they are dissolved and absorbed: they are less likely to cause irritation of the stomach lining. Claradin, Paynocil, Solprin/Disprin are soluble products; Laboprin also contains lysine.

BENORYLATE

▲ **(See table for proprietary preparations)**

- *Basic precautions:* Not suitable for those with known hypersensitivity to aspirin, with acute peptic ulceration or haemophilia. Do not take other aspirin or paracetamol drugs unwittingly.
- *Proper dosage:* 1.5 g thrice daily. Also available in suspension or granules.
- *Side effects:* Mild dyspepsia, drowsiness and rashes. If high doses are necessary dizziness, ringing in ears, deafness.
- *Special advantages:* Is superior to aspirin and paracetamol in terms of freedom from side effects.

CODEINE

(See table for formulary preparations)

- *Basic precautions:* Caution in drinking alcohol because it may enhance its effect. Caution also advised with other central-nervous system depressants, including slimming aids. Should not be taken together with MAOI antidepressants.
- *Proper dosage:* 10–60 mg taken four-hourly. Maximum dosage 200 mg daily.
- *Side effects:* Constipation and dependence.
- *Special advantages:* Constipation tends to limit its use. Is a component in many compound preparations (*see* pages 190–192).

DEXTROPROPOXYPHENE

(See table for proprietary preparations)

- *Basic precautions:* Hypersensitivity is not uncommon.
- *Proper dosage:* Depronal SA—1 capsule three to four times daily. Doloxene—1 capsule eight- to twelve-hourly.
- *Side effects:* Possible side effects include tolerance and dependence, potentiation of alcohol, impairment of mental and physical reactions, dizziness, sedation, constipation, rashes, euphoria, visual disturbances. Hazard of overdosage, especially in case of Distalgesic.
- *Special advantages:* Few in view of side effects.

DIFLUNISAL

(See table for proprietary preparations)

- *Basic precautions:* As for aspirin.
- *Proper dosage:* 500 mg twice daily; tablets to be swallowed whole, not crushed.
- *Side effects:* As for aspirin.
- *Special advantages:* Like aspirin, also has an antirheumatic effect.

DIHYDROCODEINE

(See table for proprietary preparations)

- *Basic precautions:* As for codeine. Not used if patient has severe airways obstruc-

tion, respiratory depression, or asthma. Alcohol must be avoided; reduced dosage is necessary for the elderly and those with thyroid or liver disease.
● *Proper dosage:* 30 mg taken four-hourly.
● *Side effects:* Few, but they may include constipation, gastrointestinal symptoms, headache and dizziness. Fairly high risk of habituation.
● *Special advantages:* Virtually free from sedative or hypnotic effects. Suppresses coughing.

FENOPROFEN
(See table for proprietary preparations)
● *Basic precautions:* Hypersensitivity reactions are rare. Otherwise as for aspirin; not suitable for patients with severe kidney disease. In long-term treatment routine blood testing is advisable.
● *Proper dosage:* Fenopron—300–600 mg taken four times daily. Progesic—one to two 200 mg tablets taken three to four times a day.
● *Special advantages:* Antirheumatic and analgesic.

FLUFENAMIC ACID
(See table for proprietary preparations)
● *Basic precautions:* Not suitable for patients with inflammatory bowel disease, peptic ulcer, kidney or liver disease.
● *Proper dosage:* 600 mg daily in divided doses taken with food. After four weeks dosage can usually be reduced to 400 mg daily.
● *Side effects:* As for aspirin; these usually disappear on reduced dosage.
● *Special advantages:* Antirheumatic and analgesic.

MEFENAMIC ACID
(See table for proprietary preparation)
● *Basic precautions:* As for flufenamic acid.
● *Proper dosage:* 500 mg thrice daily.
● *Side effects:* If diarrhoea occurs stop drug. Some authorities limit use of drug to seven days unless blood tests confirm that long-term treatment is safe. Other possible side effects include drowsiness, dizziness, gastrointestinal upsets, rashes, blood abnormalities.

NAPROXEN
(See table for proprietary preparations)
● *Basic precautions:* Not suitable for patients with peptic ulcer; can be used with caution and under close supervision for dyspeptics. May produce overdose effects if some sulphonamide drugs are being taken concurrently. To be used with caution for patients with kidney disease.
● *Proper dosage:* 550 mg initially, then 275 mg taken up to four times daily.
● *Side effects:* Aspirin-type side effects; occasionally swelling of hands and feet.
● *Special advantages:* Useful for management of acute pain.

PARACETAMOL
▲ ## (See table for proprietary and formulary preparations)
● *Basic precautions:* Care to be taken for long-term dosage for patients with liver or kidney disease and high blood pressure.
● *Proper dosage:* Up to 4 g daily in divided doses.

- *Side effects:* None if proper dosage is taken.
- *Special advantages:* A fairly safe painkiller.

PENTAZOCINE

(See table for proprietary preparation)

- *Basic precautions:* Not suitable for patients suffering from certain brain and skull injuries and abnormalities, or for patients being treated with other strong pain-killers, including codeine, dextropropoxyphene, dihydrocodeine, or for narcotic addicts. Care needed in cases of kidney, liver or heart disease.
- *Proper dosage:* 25–100 mg taken after meals every four hours.
- *Side effects:* Side effects are not rare; may include sedation, nausea, dizziness, sweating, skin flushes, visual disturbance, occasional hallucination. Fairly high risk of dependency.
- *Special advantages:* A powerful painkiller.

SALSALATE

(See table for proprietary preparation)

- *Basic precautions:* Not suitable for persons with kidney disease or known salicylate sensitivity. Use with caution for patients of peptic ulcer.
- *Proper dosage:* 4 capsules daily, in divided doses taken before or with food. Last dose at bedtime.
- *Side effects:* Mild aspirin-like side effects.
- *Special advantages:* Is not dissolved until it leaves stomach and so its aspirin-like action rarely creates dyspeptic problems.

SODIUM SALICYLATE

▲ (See table for proprietary preparation)

- *Basic precautions:* Not suitable for persons suffering from dyspepsia or peptic ulcer.
- *Proper dosage:* 0.5–1 g taken every four hours after meals.
- *Side effects:* As for aspirin but gastric irritation and hearing disturbances more marked.
- *Special advantages:* None.

THE MANAGEMENT OF SEVERE (GENERAL) PAIN

Sometimes one needs potent medication to give relief from severe pain. This is often done at the risk of creating a tolerance to the remedy, and thus increasing doses sometimes become necessary. There is also a risk of addiction. In many cases these risks and worries are totally irrelevant when the lifestyle and future of the patient is considered. In the control of pain in terminal malignancy the enlightened approach is to adjust both the dose and frequency of medication to make sure that the patient does not suffer pain. When the compassionate physician arranges this regime, the given dosage guides may be dramatically exceeded.

In temporarily painful conditions, for example kidney stones or gall bladder stones, powerful and prompt pain relief is seldom, if ever, followed by addiction problems. Usually the most powerful painkillers work best in the form of an injection. These are generally administered by doctors and nurses and these matters are outside the scope of this *Guide to Medicines*. They will, however, be mentioned briefly in case they become part of home management.

Preparations commonly used

BUPRENORPHINE
Temgesic
Usually given by injection, it is a long-acting painkiller and thought to have a low risk of dependency.

Temgesic sublingual
- *Basic precautions:* Care to be taken when given to patients on narcotics; may produce considerable withdrawal symptoms. Care if patients are on MAOI drugs.
- *Proper dosage:* 2 tablets to be dissolved under tongue six- to eight-hourly.
- *Side effects:* Drowsiness, affects judgement. Long duration of action.
- *Special advantages:* A new and useful painkiller, particularly for management of severe pain.

BUTORPHANOL
Stadol
- *Basic precautions:* Not to be used for patients under treatment with opiate agents, eg morphine.
- *Proper dosage:* Given by injection only.
- *Side effects:* Dizziness and nausea rarely.

DEXTROMORAMIDE
Palfium
Also available for administration by injection.
- *Basic precautions:* Not advised for use if patient is on MAOIs or within three weeks of taking such drugs. Not suitable for patients with liver disease.
- *Proper dosage:* Tablets and suppositories—5 mg, varied on instruction of doctor, up to 20 mg.
- *Side effects:* Lightheadedness, dizziness. Can be habituating.
- *Special advantages:* Powerful painkiller.

DIAMORPHINE (HEROIN)
Usually administered by injection, this is perhaps the most powerful painkiller known. It is very addictive, less likely to produce vomiting than its rival morphine. Because of its dangerous addictive qualities, however, must be administered under strict medical supervision.

DIPIPANONE
Diconal
- *Basic precautions:* Use with caution for patients with severe kidney or liver disease.
- *Proper dosage:* 1 tablet six-hourly. Very rarely increased by $\frac{1}{2}$–3 tablets a day.
- *Side effects:* Euphoria, drowsiness, blurred vision, dry mouth (rarely). Risk of habituation.
- *Special advantages:* Contains an antivomiting additive (cyclizine).

LEVORPHANOL
Dromoran
Also available for administration by injection.
- *Basic precautions:* Not suitable for patients with certain chest diseases or if MAOI drugs are being taken, or within two weeks of their withdrawal. Alcohol should be avoided.

- *Proper dosage:* 1.5–4.5 mg once or twice daily.
- *Side effects:* Nausea, vomiting, constipation, sometimes confusion.
- *Special advantages:* May be more useful than morphine in some cases.

MEPTAZINOL
Meptid
For administration by injection.
- *Basic precautions:* Not suitable for patients receiving narcotics.
- *Proper dosage:* 75–100 mg, three- to four-hourly.
- *Side effects:* Sedation, dizziness.
- *Special advantages:* Perhaps less risk of habituation, certainly less respiratory depression than caused by morphine.

METHADONE
Physeptone
Also available for administration by injection.
- *Basic precautions:* Not suitable for patients with certain chest diseases or if MAOI drugs are being taken, or within two weeks of MAOI drugs.
- *Proper dosage:* 5–10 mg, six- to eight-hourly—to be adjusted according to the degree of pain relief.
- *Side effects:* Excitement, dizziness, drowsiness, sometimes nausea and vomiting.
- *Special advantages:* An alternative to morphine, though at least as addictive. But useful for control of intractable cough.

MORPHINE
Various types of preparations available as an injection, tablets, suppositories:
Cyclimorph, Duromorph, MST Continus, Nepenthe, Morphine injection and suppository (F) and Opium tincture (F)
- *Basic precautions:* Not suitable for patients with certain chest diseases or if MAOI drugs are being taken, or within two weeks of withdrawal. Special care in use for the elderly, and those with thyroid or liver disease who may require small doses only.
- *Proper dosage:* Orally and injection—10–20 mg twice or more daily. Suppositories—15–30 mg at night.
- *Side effects:* Euphoria, a sense of mental detachment, nausea and vomiting. Duromorph has particularly strong peaking-troughing effect.
- *Special advantages:* Probably the best all-round painkiller. Cyclimorph—contains an antiemetic extra; MST Continus—(10, 30, 60 and 100 mg) are controlled-release tablets giving long-acting medication; Nepenthe—contains other papaveretum alkaloids (*see* below) and helps with sleeplessness caused by pain.

NEFOPAM
Acupan
Also available for administration by injection.
- *Basic precautions:* Not suitable for patients with convulsive disorders, heart attack, or to be taken with certain antidepressants. Not to be taken with paracetamol.
- *Proper dosage:* 30 mg, gradually increased to 90 mg, up to three times daily.
- *Side effects:* Nausea, nervousness, dry mouth.

● *Special advantages:* Non-morphine-type remedy for moderate pain which acts rapidly. Suitable for cases of chest disease patients who should not take morphine-type remedies.

PAPAVERETUM
Omnopon and papaveretum injection (F)
● *Basic precautions:* Not suitable for patients with certain chest diseases or those taking MAOI antidepressives or within two weeks of taking them. Dose reduction and special care is needed for the elderly, and in thyroid and liver disease.
● *Proper dosage:* 10–20 mg, four-hourly.
● *Side effects:* Euphoria, nausea, constipation, confusion.
● *Special advantages:* An opium preparation which contains codeine, morphine and other opium alkaloids. Also has antispasmodic effect. Useful when pain occurs in spasms and for control of acute severe skeletal-muscular pain.

PETHIDINE
Pamergan P100, Pamergan AP,
Pethilorfan (contains added levallorphan),
and Pethidine tablets and injections (F)
● *Basic precautions:* Not suitable for patients with certain chest disorders or those taking MAOI antidepressants or within two weeks of taking them. Care needed for the elderly, and in thyroid and liver disease. Pethilorfan obviates most of the respiratory problems of pethidine, but is available as an injection only and is shorter acting.
● *Proper dosage:* 50–100 mg, four-hourly.
● *Side effects:* Euphoria, dizziness, nausea, vomiting.
● *Special advantages:* Rapid action Pamergan (P100) contains an antiemetic; Pamergan AP also has antispasmodic effect. Used extensively to give relief in pain during labour.

PHENAZOCINE
Narphen
● *Basic precautions:* Not suitable for patients with convulsive disorders, delirium, thyroid disease, alcoholism, certain chest disease or in conjunction with MAOI drugs, or within two weeks of taking them. Care needed for the elderly, and for patients of kidney disease.
● *Proper dosage:* 5–20 mg, four- to six-hourly, suggested taken sublingually.
● *Side effects:* Lightheadedness, dizziness, nausea, dryness of mouth, itching; bitter taste an effect of sublingual dosage.
● *Special advantages:* Prompt and powerful painkiller whose effect lasts for five to six hours with minimal sedation. Less dependence potential than almost any other strong analgesic.

Powerful analgesic elixirs
Various elixirs (liquid preparations that are usually alcohol-based) are prescribed for chronic intractable pain. They work extraordinarily well for the control of severe pain and are used especially at home. Doctors may modify these mixtures and provide individual preparations and dosages but they are always taken only under prescription. Four commonly used, and well-tried, remedies are:

Diamorphine and cocaine elixir (Brompton cocktail)
Diamorphine, cocaine and chlorpromazine elixir
Morphine and cocaine elixir
Morphine, cocaine and chlorpromazine elixir
Dosages of all the above are variable and suggested by the prescribing physician.

Migraine remedies

Migraine is a curious disease characterised by headache, visual disturbances and vomiting. It is probable that it is basically due to changes occurring in certain arteries inside the brain. Migraine management can involve prophylaxis (prevention) and actual treatment of attacks.

MIGRAINE PREVENTION

Prevention is usually only thought feasible for patients who have more than one attack per month. Medical prophylaxis and treatment of migraine is an area where rapid changes are taking place and several new remedies are being evaluated. So much so that patients may find themselves using new migraine preparations which have not been detailed in this book.

Preparations commonly used

CLONIDINE
Dixarit

- *Basic precautions:* May be unsuitable for depressive patients. Care needed if patient is under treatment for hypertension as effect of antihypertensive may be increased.
- *Proper dosage:* 2 tablets twice daily; if no response is evident in two weeks, increase to 3 tablets twice daily.
- *Side effects:* May lower blood pressure and produce dizziness. An effective prophylactic for many patients. Treatment must be withdrawn gradually. Impotence a common side effect.

METHYSERGIDE
Deseril

- *Basic precautions:* Not suitable for patients with artery or vein disease, inflammatory conditions, kidney, heart, or liver disease, high blood pressure and certain chest diseases. One drug-free interval of a month for every six months of treatment is recommended.
- *Proper dosage:* 1–2 mg nocturnally, then taken with meals two to three times daily according to response. Start with 1 tablet at bedtime, increase over a two-week period to optimum dose. Aim to find lowest dose that will control most of the attacks (or perhaps 75 per cent of them). Gradually 'tail off' treatment towards the end of six months. Special care should be exercised and be alert for loin, flank, or chest pain or coldness of limbs and numbness while taking the drug. Chest and heart examinations by doctor at regular intervals is recommended. If any of above problems develop medication should be stopped.
- *Side effects:* Possible side effects include nausea, abdominal discomfort, dizziness,

drowsiness, leg swelling, insomnia, cramps, rashes, hair loss. Rare side effects may be tissue and lung fibrosis and artery spasm.

- *Special advantages:* Will prevent or reduce severe migraines in 60–70 per cent of cases. The side effects, however, can be worrying, so this remedy is usually reserved for severe, intractable migraine.

PIZOTIFEN

Sanomigran

- *Basic precautions:* May produce drowsiness, so driving and machinery operation are hazards. Not suitable for patients with closed-angle glaucoma, or for male patients with urinary problems.
- *Proper dosage:* Two strengths of tablets—0.5 and 1.5 mg. Dosage—1.5 mg tablet at night; or 0.5 mg three times daily.
- *Side effects:* Drowsiness, dry mouth, weight gain, nausea and muscle pain.
- *Special advantages:* A useful remedy working centrally in the brain to reduce the artery distension associated with migraine. Also prevents 'cluster headaches'.

PROCHLORPERAZINE

See Chapter 17: Remedies controlling nausea.

PROPRANOLOL

See under non-barbiturate drugs used as tranquillisers, page 154.

MIGRAINE TREATMENTS

Many migraines respond to simple or compound analgesics, especially aspirin and paracetamol (*see* pages 178 and 180). Soluble and effervescent preparations are particularly helpful as are those containing antiemetics. When these fail, ergotamine (a derivative of the ergot fungus) remedies are often used and have to be carefully monitored for side effects.

Proprietary compound and non-ergotamine remedies
These are a mixed bag of remedies.

▲ Migraleve
Tablets of two colours containing analgesics (paracetamol and codeine), an anti-nauseant (buclizine) and a surface laxative (dioctylsodium sulphosuccinate) to prevent the constipating effects of codeine.

- *Basic precautions:* Long-term treatment needs supervision if patient has kidney disease. The antihistamine (antiemetic) in the pink tablets may cause drowsiness and make driving/machinery minding a hazard.
- *Proper dosage:* 2 pink tablets immediately on commencement of, or prior to, attack (if warning precedes symptoms). If symptoms persist, 2 yellow tablets, taken three-hourly. Maximum dosage: 2 pink and 6 yellow tablets per twenty-four hours.
- *Side effects:* Rare drowsiness.
- *Special advantages:* A useful non-ergotamine remedy which is therapeutically well designed and virtually free from side effects.

Migravess
Contains aspirin as its analgesic, together with metoclopramide, an antiemetic substance that hastens gastric emptying and probably absorption of the analgesic.

- *Basic precautions:* Care to be exercised in use by the young and elderly.
- *Proper dosage:* 2 tablets dissolved in half a glass of water at first signs of attack, repeated to maximum of 3 doses per day.
- *Side effects:* Spasm of facial muscles or neck muscles occurs rarely. May cause drowsiness in rare cases.
- *Special advantages:* An effective non-ergotamine remedy.

Paramax

This remedy is similar to Migravess except that paracetamol is the analgesic rather than aspirin (in powder or tablet form).

- *Basic precautions:* As for Migravess.
- *Proper dosage:* 2 (tablets or sachets) at first warning of attack, repeated to a maximum of 6 tablets in twenty-four-hour period.
- *Side effects:* As for Migravess.
- *Special advantages:* Paracetamol is less irritating to the stomach than aspirin, although it is not quite such a powerful analgesic.

Midrid

Contains a blood vessel 'stabiliser' (isometheptene), a sedative (dichloralphenazone) and a painkiller (paracetamol).

- *Basic precautions:* Not suitable for patients with severe kidney, liver, heart or hypertensive disease, or glaucoma, or for patients on MAOI therapy.
- *Proper dosage:* 2 capsules at once on occurrence of attack, then 1–2 capsules taken four-hourly; maximum 8 per day.
- *Side effects:* Dizziness.
- *Special advantages:* For suitable patients an excellent migraine remedy, in many ways a halfway-house between the other remedies in this group and ergotamine remedies.

The ergotamine migraine remedies

Ergotamine is reserved for patients who do not respond to other remedies. It is highly specific against some migraines, but is limited in its use because the side effects occur frequently and can be dangerous unless treatment is discontinued. In some patients repeated use seems to promote a state of dependence in which withdrawal of the drug precipitates 'withdrawal' migraine. Ergotamine treatments should never be considered as a prophylactic or be repeated at intervals of less than four days.

Cafergot

Available in two forms, tablets and suppositories, both containing ergotamine and caffeine.

Tablets

- *Basic precautions:* Not suitable for patients with disease of arteries, kidney or liver, porphyria, septic conditions and high blood pressure. Stop treatment immediately if weakness of legs, muscle pain, tingling and numbness occur.
- *Proper dosage:* 2 tablets at first warning of attack, plus 1 tablet half an hour later (if necessary) and repeated at half-hour intervals until a maximum of 6 is taken. Subsequently, the total dose found to be effective is taken at once. Maximum tablets 6 per day or 10 per week.

- *Side effects:* These include nausea, vomiting, muscle pain, numbness and tingling. There is some risk of dependency with the suppositories.
- *Special advantages:* Will cure 80 per cent of migraine headaches.

Suppositories
- *Basic precautions:* As for tablets.
- *Proper usage:* 1 suppository to be used at first sign of attack. Repeat if necessary. Maximum 3 suppositories per day, or 5 per week.
- *Side effects:* As for tablets, plus drowsiness.
- *Special advantages:* Useful for those in whom vomiting is part of migraine and who tend to vomit oral remedies.

Dihydergot

Tablet, oral solution and injectable form. This is a chemically modified ergotamine (dihydroergotamine mesylate) that has less worrying side effects than the sister compound. It is the only ergotamine preparation that may be considered to be a prophylactic. It is also less effective than ergotamine in its action.
- *Basic precautions:* No special precautions necessary for oral preparations.
- *Proper dosage:* 2–3 tablets or 20–30 drops, repeated half-hourly if necessary. Maximum dosage 10 tablets or 100 drops daily.
- *Side effects:* Nausea and vomiting.
- *Special advantages:* In oral form Dihydergot is a reasonably safe ergotamine-type preparation.

Lingraine—sublingual tablet
- *Basic precautions:* As for Cafergot.
- *Proper dosage:* 1 (2 mg) tablet dissolved under tongue at first sign of attack, repeated in half an hour. Maximum dosage 3 tablets per day, 6 per week.
- *Side effects:* As for Cafergot.
- *Special advantages:* An 'ergotamine only' preparation with no complicating factors introduced by other medicaments. Safe if properly used.

Migril

A combination of ergotamine, with antiemetic (cyclizine) and caffeine.
- *Basic precautions:* As for Cafergot. It may cause sedation so care is needed if driving and operating machinery.
- *Proper dosage:* 1–2 tablets taken at first warning of attack, then $\frac{1}{2}$–1 tablet half-hourly. Maximum dosage 4 tablets per attack, 6 tablets per week.
- *Side effects:* As for Cafergot but also causes sedation.
- *Special advantages:* Has the potency of ergotamine remedies and an antiemetic effect.

Remedies used for trigeminal neuralgia

Many of the general analgesics may be prescribed for this unpleasant illness, which causes pain in the head and face. But there is a specific remedy for this available—carbamazepine. This drug is also used in epilepsy (*see* page 171).

Remedies commonly used

CARBAMAZEPINE
Tegretol
- *Basic precautions:* Special care to be taken in some heart conditions. May reduce effectiveness of contraceptive pill unless a higher dose pill is used. Not suitable for use with, or within two weeks of MAOI treatment.
- *Proper dosage:* 100 mg daily (tablets) or 5 ml syrup, increasing until response is obtained. Most patients respond to a maximum of 200 mg four times daily. To be used as treatment for an acute condition, not as a prophylactic.
- *Side effects:* Possible side effects include dizziness, double vision, dry mouth, diarrhoea and, rarely, nausea. Severe rashes.
- *Special advantages:* A useful addition to possible treatments for a nasty and painful illness.

Remedies for pain arising in the urinary tract

Urinary pain has special characteristics. Treatment of the cause (in the case of infection) combats the pain in the best possible way. Ordinary analgesics, however, have an important part to play. But there are a few particular remedies that are useful when general remedies fail.

EMEPRONIUM
Cetiprin
This increases the bladder capacity and delays the urge to empty bladder. It is used in diseases in which pain associated with the bladder occurs, in undue frequency in passing of urine, or for incontinence in the elderly.
- *Basic precautions:* Not suitable for patients who find swallowing difficult, or sufferers of prostate disease which has produced a distended bladder. Patients should not lie down within ten to fifteen minutes of taking tablets. Caution needed in use by patients with glaucoma or stomach trouble or inflammatory gut disorders, such as Crohn's disease.
- *Proper dosage:* Up to 200 mg thrice daily or 200–400 mg at night taken with at least 100 ml of water.
- *Side effects:* Rarely, dry mouth, or ulceration of the gullet if tablets not swallowed as directed.

PHENAZOPYRIDINE
▲ Pyridium
- *Basic precautions:* Not suitable for patients with liver disease, kidney failure, coeliac disease or gluten sensitivity. Colours urine red.
- *Proper dosage:* 2 tablets thrice daily before meals.
- *Side effects:* Gastrointestinal upset, headache, dizziness. Anaemia is a rare side effect.
- *Special advantages:* Useful for urinary tract pain of all types.

FLAVOXATE
Urispas

- *Basic precautions:* Not suitable for patients with obstructive problems of the stomach, duodenum, elsewhere in bowel or in urinary tract. Care advised for persons with glaucoma.
- *Proper dosage:* 2 tablets thrice daily.
- *Side effects:* Rarely—headache, nausea, fatigue, diarrhoea, blurred vision, dry mouth.
- *Special advantages:* Useful for relieving symptomatic bladder pain (cystitis), urethritis, prostatitis.

Compound analgesics

This section consists of a large number of prescription and OTC remedies. The basic precautions, proper dosage and side effects can, in most cases, be deduced from their components.

General note: All of these drugs are in tablet form unless stated otherwise.

Compound name	Components
▲ Anadin	Aspirin, caffeine, quinine sulphate
▲ Anadin Soluble	Aspirin, caffeine
▲ Anadin Maximum Strength	Aspirin (500 mg), caffeine
▲ Antoin Dispersible Tablets	Aspirin, codeine phosphate, caffeine citrate
▲ Aspirin and Codeine	Aspirin and codeine phosphate (tablets and dispersible effervescent base)
▲ Beecham's Powders	Caffeine, aspirin, salicylamide, cinnamon oil (tablets and powder)
▲ Cafadol	Paracetamol, caffeine
Carisoma Co	Carisoprodol, paracetamol, caffeine
▲ Codanin	Codeine, paracetamol
▲ Codeine and Paracetamol	Codeine phosphate, paracetamol
▲ Codis Dispersible Tablets	Aspirin, codeine phosphate
▲ Codural	Paracetamol, caffeine, homatropin
▲ Cogene	Aspirin, codeine, caffeine
▲ Cosalgesic	Dextropropoxyphene hydrochloride, paracetamol
Delimon	Morazone hydrochloride, paracetamol, salicylamide
Dihydrocodeine and Paracetamol	Dihydrocodeine tartrate, paracetamol (500 mg)
Distalgesic	Dextropropoxyphene hydrochloride, paracetamol
Distalgesic Soluble	Dextropropoxyphene napsylate, paracetamol

Compound name	Components
▲ Doan's Backache Pills	Paracetamol, sodium salicylate, aloin
Dolasan (Lilly)	Dextropropoxyphene napsylate, aspirin
Doloxene Compound	Dextropropoxyphene napsylate, aspirin
▲ E.P. Tablets	Paracetamol, caffeine, codeine
Equagesic	Ethoheptazine citrate, meprobamate, aspirin
▲ Femerital	Ambucetamide, paracetamol
▲ Feminax	Paracetamol, salicylamide, codeine
Fortagesic	Pentazocine hydrochloride, paracetamol
▲ Hedex Seltzer	Paracetamol, caffeine
▲ Hypon	Aspirin, caffeine, codeine phosphate
Lobak	Chlormezanone, paracetamol
▲ Medocodene	Paracetamol, codeine phosphate
▲ Myolgin Dispersible Tablets	Paracetamol, aspirin, codeine phosphate, caffeine citrate, acetomenaphthone
Napsalgesic	Dextropropoxyphene napsylate, aspirin
▲ Neurodol	Paracetamol, caffeine
▲ Neurodyne	Paracetamol, codeine phosphate (capsules)
Norgesic	Orphenadrine citrate, paracetamol
Onadox-118	Aspirin, dihydrocodeine tartrate (dispersible tablets)
Paedo-Sed	Dichloralphenazone, paracetamol (syrup)
▲ Panadeine Co	Corresponds to codeine and paracetamol tablets
▲ Paracodol	Paracetamol, codeine phosphate (dispersible tablets)
▲ Paradeine	Paracetamol, codeine phosphate, phenolphthalein
▲ Parahypon	Paracetamol, codeine phosphate, caffeine
▲ Parake	Paracetamol, codeine phosphate
▲ Paralgin	Paracetamol, caffeine, codeine phosphate
Paramol-118	Corresponds to dihydrocodeine and paracetamol tablets
Parazolidin	Phenylbutazone, paracetamol
▲ Pardale	Paracetamol, codeine phosphate, caffeine hydrate
Paxidal	Paracetamol, meprobamate, caffeine
▲ Pharmidone	Codeine phosphate, diphenhydramine hydrochloride, paracetamol, caffeine

Table continues on next page

Compound Analgesics *continued*

Compound name	Components
▲ Phensic	Aspirin, caffeine
▲ Propain	Codeine phosphate, diphenhydramine hydrochloride, paracetamol, caffeine
Robaxisal Forte	Methocarbamol, aspirin
▲ Safapryn	Paracetamol, aspirin
▲ Safapryn Co	Paracetamol, codeine phosphate, aspirin
▲ Solpadeine	Paracetamol, codeine phosphate, caffeine (dispersible tablets)
Syndol	Paracetamol, codeine phosphate, doxylamine succinate, caffeine
Tandalgesic	Oxyphenbutazone, paracetamol
Trancoprin	Aspirin, chlormezanone
▲ Unigesic	Paracetamol, caffeine (capsules)
▲ Veganin	Corresponds to aspirin, paracetamol and codeine tablets
▲ Yeast Vite	Salicylamide, caffeine, yeast, vitamin B
Zactipar	Ethoheptazine citrate, paracetamol
Zactirin	Ethoheptazine citrate, aspirin

Appendix

DRUG INTERACTION

When you think about it even superficially, interaction between drugs must occur. A drug that, say, damps down peristaltic activity like propantheline will naturally be antagonistic to a drug like metoclopramide that works by increasing the propulsive waves that pass through an organ. In a way, one is an antidote to another.

There is another type of drug interaction which gives cause for concern. This occurs when one medicine alters the absorption, distribution or the excretion of another. Or even the rate at which the body breaks it down into inactive components. Again one drug may have a sort of chemical affinity to another and binds itself to it in such a way chemically that it cannot exert its full strength of action. An example of this occurs with the Pill. Some sedatives and antibiotics inhibit the effectiveness of the Pill in this way and women find themselves pregnant.

Such effects are not usually predictable and many are discovered quite by accident. Usually, and this complicates the matter, only a relatively small proportion of the total number of patients potentially at risk because of such drug interaction, actually suffer from it. In other words, idiosyncrasy is a factor in drug interaction and one that cannot always be quantified when treatment schedules are arranged.

In an ideal world one would hope that your GP would stress these possible snags, but unfortunately you cannot always count on this happening.

If you are taking	*Do not take*	*Possible effect if you do*
I **Drugs used to constrict blood vessels** (*see* especially those used in Chapter 14, nose and throat)	Insulin and other hypoglycaemics	Can potentiate hypertensive crises
Adrenaline and noradrenaline	Tricyclic and MAOI antidepressants	
	Beta-blockers used in cases of heart disease (consult your doctor)	Cause rise in blood pressure

If you are taking	Do not take	Possible effect if you do
II Painkillers (see Chapter 16)		
Aspirin-containing remedies	Metoclopramide	Increase effect
Diflunisal	Antacids Indigestion remedies	Reduce effect
Naproxen	Probenecid	Increased blood levels of Naproxen accumulate, increase effects/side effects
Paracetamol	Cholestyramine Metoclopramide	Reduce effect Increase effect
III Sleeping pills, sedatives generally	Alcohol, antidepressants, antihistamines, narcotic painkillers	Increase action
IV Antidepressants (see Chapter 15)		
(a) Tricyclic antidepressants	Alcohol	Produces increased sedation
(b) MAOI antidepressants	Sympathomimetic amines (cold remedies), ephedrine, femcamfamin, femfluramine, levodopa, oxypertine	Sudden rise of blood pressure, up to two weeks after stopping MAOI
	Pethidine, reserpine, tricyclic antidepressants	Excitation, high blood pressure
V Drugs used for epilepsy (see Chapter 15)		
(a) General epilepsy remedies	Antidepressants, phenothiazines Oral contraceptives	Reduce effect of anticonvulsants Causes fluid retention which may precipitate fits in epileptics under medication
(b) Especially:		
(i) Phenobarbitone, primidone	Phenytoin, sodium valproate	Increase sedation
(ii) Phenytoin	Chloramphenicol, co-trimoxazole, diazepam, dicoumarol, disulfiram, isoniazid, pheneturide, phenylbutazone, sulphaphenazole, sulthiame, viloxazine	Increase effect
	Sodium valproate	Transient increased effect
(c) Sodium valproate	Carbamazepine, phenobarbitone, phenytoin, primidone	Reduce effect
VI Drugs used for Parkinson's disease and other nervous disorders (see Chapter 15)		
(a) Anticholinergic-type remedies (see Chapter 15)	Amantadine, disopyramide, antihistamines and phenothiazine drugs Tricyclic/MAOI antidepressants, antihypertensives, methyldopa, orphenadrine and sympathomimetics	Increase dry mouth, urine-retention problems and confusion All potentially hazardous combined with anticholinergics
(b) Levodopa	Chlordiazepoxide, diazepam Pyridoxine Metoclopramide	Reduce therapeutic effect Reduce therapeutic effect Increase therapeutic effect

If you are taking	Do not take	Possible effect if you do
VI Drugs used for Parkinson's disease and other nervous disorders *continued*		
(c) The phenothiazines	Metoclopramide	Increase side effects
(d) Haloperidol	Metoclopramide	Increase side effects
(e) Lithium carbonate	Diuretics, any drug which reduces sodium in body, diclofenac, indomethacin, phenylbutazone	Increase action
	Aminophylline	Increases renal excretions
VII The Pill	Some antibiotics, barbiturates, carbamazepine, dichloralphenazone, phenytoin, primidone	Reduce efficacy
VIII Drugs used for rheumatism (*see* Chapter 11)		
(a) Indomethacin	Probenecid	Increase action
(b) Penicillamine	Iron tablets, zinc sulphate	Reduce action
(c) Phenylbutazone	Cholestyramine	Reduce action
(d) Probenecid	Aspirin	Reduce action
	Dapsone (anti-malarial)	Increase side effects
(e) Sulphinpyrazone	Do not take pyrazinamide	Reduces action
IX Drugs used to combat infection (*see* Chapter 4)		
(a) Amioglycoside antibiotics	Ethacrynic acid, frusemide	Increase side effects
(b) The tetracycline antibiotics generally	Antacids, iron tablets, zinc sulphate	Reduce effect
Doxycycline	Barbiturates, carbamazepine, phenytoin	Reduce effect
(c) Furazolidone, metronidazole	Alcohol	Emetic reaction
(d) Griseofulvin	Phenobarbitone	Decrease effect
(e) Lincomycin	Kaolin mixtures	Decrease effect
(f) Nitrofurantoin	Probenecid	Increase effect
(g) Phenoxymethyl penicillin	Neomycin	Reduce effect
X Thyroxine (thyroid replacement) (*see* Chapter 5)	Cholestryramine	Reduce effect
	Fenclofenac, phenylbutazone, phenytoin	Gives false (biochemical) blood levels

GENERAL INDEX

Acne 76, 89–93
Adrenalin 23
Allergies
  chest illnesses 37–8, 48
  eyes 136, 141
  skin problems 76, 88
  tranquillisers 154
  see also Sensitivity reactions
Anaemia 117–22
Analgesics, see Painkillers
Antacids 18, 19–20, 21, 194
Antibiotics 58–63
  acne 89
  skin infections 81
Anticholinergics 22, 23–4, 39, 44–5, 132
Antidepressants 160–6
Antihistamines 48, 87, 95, 132, 133, 148
Anti-itch preparations 87–9
Antiseptics 79–81
Antispasmodics 19, 21, 22, 23–5
Antithyroid drugs 74–5
Antiviral drugs 70–1
Appetite suppressants 53–7
Arthritis 123
Artificial sweeteners 57
Asthma 38–49
  bronchodilators 38–45
  prevention 48–9
  steroids 45–8
Athlete's foot 81, 83

Barbiturates 153, 158–9
Barrier creams 86
Barrier devices (contraceptives) 111
Blood pressure 13
Boils 76, 81
Bowels 14, 22
  surgery medication 29

British National Formulary 49
Bronchiectasis 37
Bronchitis 38, 39, 44
Bronchodilators 38–45
Bronchospasm (wheezing) 38–49

Calluses 93–5
Cancer
  lung 37
  pain relief 181
  skin 85
Cap, cervical 111
Cephalosporins 58, 61
Cervix 99
Chest illnesses 37–52
Choreas 176
Children 13
Cholinergics 23
Colon disorders 34–6
Colds 146
Condoms 109
Constipation 29–34
Contraception 109–16
Contraceptive Pill, see Pill
Corneal ulceration 136, 138
Corns 76, 93–5
Corticosteroids 95
Co-trimoxazole 58, 64
Cough mixtures 49–52
Cretinism 73
Crohn's disease 26
Cystitis 190

Dandruff 77
Depression 160–6
Dermatitis 76, 77, 95
Diabetics 13, 195
  cough mixtures 52
Diaphragm (contraceptive) 111
Diaphragm (midriff) 17
Diarrhoea 22, 26–9

Diverticulitis 22, 26
Dizziness 134–5
Doctors and patients 10–12
Dopamine 174
Dumas vault device 111
Dyspepsia 18–20

Ears 144–6
Eczema 76, 77, 95–7
Elixirs 52, 184
Encephalitis 174
Endocrine glands 45
Enemas 35–6
Enzyme treatments
  rheumatism 131
Epilepsy 169–74, 194
Exercise 54
Expectorants 50–1
Eyes 136–43

Fibrositis 123
Focal epilepsy 171–3
Food poisoning 26
Fungus infections 67–70, 99
  skin 81, 83–5

Gall bladder stones 181
Gastric acid 21
Gastrointestinal spasm 22–5
Gastrointestinal tract 14, 26
Giddiness 132, 134–5
Gingivitis 15–16
Glaucoma 136, 138, 141
Goitre 72–3
Gout 123, 129–30
Grand mal 170, 171–3
Gullet (oesophagus) 17–18
Gums 15–16

H₂ receptor blocking agents 21
Heart disease 13
Hepatitis, infective 70

Herpes simplex virus 138
Hiatus hernia 17–18
Hookworms 107, 108
Hormonal contraception 111–16
Hormone Replacement Therapy (HRT) 101–2
Hypersexuality 104
Hypofertility 99

Impetigo 81
Impotence 98, 104
Infection
  asthma 37–8, 48
  control of 58–71, 195–6
  eyes 136–41
  skin 81–3
Infertility 98–100
Influenza (flu) 70, 149–50
Intertrigo 76
Intestines 22
Iodine 72
Iron composition
  anaemia treatment 118–19
Iron replacement therapy 117–18

Kidney stones 181

Labyrinthitis 134
Laxatives 29–34
Linctuses 50, 51–2
Lung diseases 37

Mania 160, 165, 166–7
Manic-depression 159, 160, 167
MAOI antidepressants 164, 193, 194
Megaloblastic anaemia 117
Ménières disease 134
Menopause 100–3
Metabolism 72
Migraine 185–9
Motion sickness 132–3
Mouth 14–17, 150–2
  fungal infections 68–70, 150–1
  ulcers 16–17
Mouthwashes 15–16, 151–2
'Mussel' cures for rheumatism 131
Myoclonic jerks 170, 173
Myxoedema 73

Nasal congestion 147–8
Nausea 132–4
Nerves 153–76
Nervous system 38–9, 76
Neuralgia 188–9
Nose 146–9

Oesophagus (gullet) 17–18
Oestrogen 101–3, 111, 112

Oral contraceptives, see Pill, contraceptive
Otitis 145–6
Ovaries 100

Pain control 177–92
Painkillers 177–92, 194
  for rheumatism 125–9
Parkinsonism 174–6
Parkinson's disease 174–5, 194–5
Penicillins 58, 59–60
Peptic ulcers 16, 18–22
Peristalsis 22
Petit mal 170, 173
Phobias 159
Pill, contraceptive 111–16, 193, 195
  combined-Pill 112–15
  progestogen-only 115–16
Pleurisy 37
Pneumonia 37
Poliomyelitis (polio) 70
Porphyria 86
Pregnancy
  anaemia 119–20
  epilepsy 170, 171
  sickness 133
Pre-meal aids 56
Progestogen 102, 111, 112, 115–16
Pruritis 34
Psoriasis 76, 95–7
Psychoneuroses 159
Psychosis 159–69
Pyloric stenosis 19
Pyorrhoea 15

Rabies 70
Rectum disorders 34–6
Replacement meals 57
Rheumatism 123–31, 195
Ringworm 83
Roundworms 106, 108
Rubella 70

Schizophrenia 159, 167–9
Sebaceous glands 76
Sebum 89
Sedatives 95, 153–9, 194
Sensitivity reactions
  antibiotics 59, 61, 63
  see also Allergies
Sexual dysfunction 98–104
Sexual problems 103–4
Shampoos 77–9
Skin 76–97
  acne 76, 89–93
  camouflage 87
  cancer 85
  cleaners 77–9
  infections 81–3
  fungus 67–70, 81, 83–5
  protection 85–7
Sleeping tablets 153–9, 194

Slimming aids 53–7
Smallpox 70
Spastic bowel syndrome 22, 26
Spermicides 110
Spots 81, see also Acne
Steroids
  acne 89
  asthma 45–8
  diarrhoea 27–8
  eye infections 138–9
  rectal disorders 35–6
  skin diseases 96–7
Stomach 18–25
Stress
  chest illnesses 37–8, 48
  skin problems 76, 89
Sulphonamides 58, 64–6, 72
Sunburn 85
Sun-screeners 85–7
Suppositories 33, 35–6
Sympathomimetics 23, 38–45, 147, 148

Tapeworms 107–8
Tearless eyes 143
Testosterone 98, 103
Tetracyclines 58, 61–3, 85, 89, 93
Threadworms 105–6, 108
Throat 150
Thrush 61, 150
Thyroid gland 72–5
  hormone deficiency disease 72–3
  overaction 73
Tics 176
Tinea 81
Tranquillisers 153–7
Trichomonas 99
Tricyclic antidepressants 104, 160–4, 193, 194
Trigeminal neuralgia 188–9
Tuberculosis 63, 66–7

Ulcerative colitis 26
Ulcer-healing drugs 19, 21–2
Ulcers
  mouth 16–17
  peptic 16, 18–22
Urinary tract 65–6
  189–90

Vagina
  fungal infections 68–70, 99
Vertigo 132, 134–5
Vimule 111
Viruses 70–1
Vomiting 132–4

Warts 76, 93–5
Wax in ears 144
Wheezing 38–49
Worms 105–8

Xanthine bronchodilators 44–5

LIST AND INDEX OF DRUGS

In the following list of drugs, those in SMALL CAPITALS represent the principal ingredients active in commercial preparations. These generic drugs and their derivative proprietary and formulary preparations (represented in ordinary type here) will be found on the pages indicated.

After the names of all proprietary and formulary drugs, you will find the symbols **P**, **▲**, or both. **P** indicates that a preparation is available on prescription; **▲** that it is OTC (available over-the-counter); **P**+**▲** that it is both. This latter reference may be of use, both from a point of view of information and because, with costs running at £1.40 a prescription, over-the-counter rates for the same drug could prove competitive.

ACEPIFYLLINES 45
ACETARSOL 16, 151
ACETAZOLAMIDE 141
ACETIC ACID 94
Acetoxyl (P+▲) 91
Achromycin (P) 62, 83, 137, 145
Acnegel (P+▲) 91
Acnil (P+▲) 90
Acriflex (▲) 79
Actal (P+▲) 20
Actidil (P) 149
Actifed Compound Linctus (P+▲) 52
Actifed Expectorant (P+▲) 50
Actifed tablets (P+▲) 148
Actinac (P) 92
Actonorm gel (P+▲) 20
    powder and tablets (P) 25
Actonorm-Sed (P) 25
Acupan (P) 183–4
ACYCLOVIR 70, 71, 137, 138
Adcortyl (P) 47, 97
Adcortyl in Orabase (P) 16
ADRENALINE 142
Adrenaline and atropine spray (F) (P) 42
ADRENALINE-TYPE 41–2
Afrazine (P+▲) 147
Agarol (P+▲) 30
Agiolax (P+▲) 31
Akineton (P) 176
Albucid (P) 137
Alcopar (P+▲) 106
Alcos-Anal (P+▲) 35
Aleudrin tablets (P) 42
Algesal (P+▲) 124
ALGINATES AND ANTACIDS 18
ALGINATES AND CARBENOXOLONE AND ANTACIDS 18
Algipan (P+▲) 124
Algispray (▲) 125
Alka-Seltzer (▲) 178
Allegron (P) 161, 163
ALLOPURINOL 129–30
ALOES 34
Alophen Pills (P+▲) 34

ALPAZOLAM 154
Alphaderm (P) 96
Alphosyl (P+▲) 78
Alrheumat (P) 126
Altacite (P+▲) 20
Altacite plus (P+▲) 20
Alu-Cap (P+▲) 19
Aludrox (P+▲) 19
Aludrox SA (P) 25
Aluhyde (P) 25
ALUMINIUM 91
ALUMINIUM ACETATE 145
Aluminium acetate ear drops (F) (P+▲) 145
ALUMINIUM HYDROXIDE 19
Aluminium hydroxide mixture and tablets (F) (P+▲) 19
ALUMINIUM PHOSPHATE 19
Alupent (P) 43
Alupent Expectorant (P) 50
Aluphos (P+▲) 19
ALVERINE 23
AMANTADINE 70, 71, 174, 194
Amesec (P) 43
Amfipen (P) 59
AMINOBENZOIC ACID 86
Aminobenzoic acid lotion (F) (P+▲) 86
AMINOPHYLLINE 45
Aminophylline (F) (P+▲) 45
AMITRIPTYLINE 160, 161
Amitriptyline (F) (P) 160, 161
Ammonium and Ipecacuanha mixture (F) (P+▲) 50
Ammonium chloride mixture (F) (P+▲) 50
Ammonium chloride and morphine mixture (F) (P+▲) 50
Amoxil (P) 59
AMOXYCILLIN 59
AMPHETAMINE (DEXAMPHETA-MINE) 55
AMPHOTERICIN 68, 83, 151
AMPICILLIN 59
Ampicillin (F) (P) 59
Ampiclox (P) 60
AMYLOBARBITONE 158

Amylobarbitone (F) (P) 158
Amytal (P) 158
Anacal (P) 36
Anadin (▲) 190
Anadin Maximum Strength (▲) 190
Anadin Soluble (▲) 190
Anaflex (P+▲) 82, 151
Anafranil (P) 160, 162
Ananase Forte (P) 131
Anbesol (P+▲) 17
Ancoloxin (P+▲) 133
Andrew's Liver Salts (▲) 33
Androcur (P) 104
Andursil (P+▲) 20
Anestan (▲) 43
Anodesyn (P+▲) 35
Anorvit tablets (▲) 120
Anovlar 21 (P) 112
Anquil (P) 168
Antasil (P+▲) 20
Antepar (▲) 105
Anthisan (P+▲) 149
ANTHRAQUINONE 151
ANTHRAQUINONE AND SALICYLIC ACID 17
Antistin-Privine (P+▲) 147
Antoin Dispersible tablets (▲) 190
Anturan (P) 130
Antussin (▲) 51
Anugesic-HC (P) 36
Anusol (P+▲) 35
Anusol HC (P) 36
Anxon (P) 155–6
Apisate (P) 55
APP consolidated (P) 25
Apsin VK (P) 60
Aquadrate (P+▲) 96
Aqueous iodine solution (P) 74
ARACHIS OIL 33
ARACHIS OIL/LIQUID PARAFFIN 77
Aradolene (P+▲) 124
Argotone (P+▲) 147
Arobon (P+▲) 27
Aromatic chalk and opium powder (F) (P) 26

Artane (P) 176
Artracin (P) 127
Asilone (P+▲) 20
Asmapax (P) 43
Asma-Vydrin (P+▲) 44
Aspellin (P+▲) 124, 125
Aspergum (P+▲) 178
ASPIRIN 125, 178–9, 194, 195
Aspirin (F) (P+▲) 178
Aspirin Dispersible (F) (P+▲)
   178
Aspirin and Codeine (P+▲) 190
Aspro (▲) 178
Aspro Clear (▲) 178
Atarax (P) 155
Atensine (P) 155
Ativan (P) 156
ATROPINE 23, 132
ATROPINE AND DEPTROPINE 44
Atropine Methonitrate and
   sulphate (F) (P) 44
Atropine sulphate (F) (P) 23
   tablets (F) (P) 132
Atrovent (P) 44
Audax (P+▲) 145
Audicort (P) 145, 146
Audinorm (P+▲) 144
Augmentin (P) 59
Auralgicin (P+▲) 146
Auraltone (P+▲) 146
Aureomycin (P) 62, 137
Aventyl (P) 161, 163
Avloclor (P) 128
Avomine (P+▲) 133
Avrogel (P+▲) 90, 94
Ayds (▲) 56
Ayrton's corn and wart paint
   (P+▲) 94
AZAPROPAZONE 125
AZATADINE 148

Bactrim (P) 64, 65
Balmosa (P+▲) 124
Banistyl (P) 149
Bayolin (P+▲) 124
BC 500 with Iron Tablets
   (P+▲) 120
BECLOMETHASONE AND BETA-
   METHASONE 46
Beconase (P) 147
Becotide (P) 46
Beecham's Pills (P) 34
Beecham's Powders (▲) 190
   Hot Lemon (▲) 150
   Mentholated (▲) 150
Bellocarb (P) 25
Benadryl (P+▲) 133, 149
Benafed (P+▲) 52, 148
Benemid (P) 130
Bengue's Balsam and SG (P+▲)
   24
Benoral (P+▲) 178
BENORYLATE 178, 179
Benoxyl (P+▲) 91
BENPERIDOL 168, 169
Benylin Day and Night (▲)
   150
Benylin Expectorant (P+▲) 50
Benylin Fortified (▲) 51
Benylin with Codeine (P) 51
BENZALKONIUM 79, 94
BENZATHINE PENICILLIN 59
BENZHEXOL 176
Benzhexol (F) (P) 176

BENZOCAINE AND CETYLPYRIDIUM
   16
BENZOCTAMINE 154
BENZOIC ACID 83
BENZOYL PEROXIDE 91
BENZTROPINE 176
BENZYDAMINE 151
BENZYLPENICILLIN 59
BEPHENIUM 106
Bephenium (P+▲) 107
Berkdopa (P) 175
Berkmycen (P) 62
Berkolol (P) 156–7
Berkomine (P) 161, 162
Berotec (P) 39
Betadine (P+▲) 80
   Mouth Wash (P+▲) 152
BETAHISTINE 135
BETAMETHASONE 35, 46, 47, 97,
   138, 145
Betnelan (P) 47
Betnesol (P) 47, 138, 145, 147
Betnesol-N (P) 145, 147
Betnovate (P) 35, 97
Betresol-N (P) 139
Bextasol (P) 46
Biactol (▲) 93
Bidrolar (P+▲) 31
Bile Beans (P) 34
Bi Novum (P) 112
Biogastrone (P) 21, 22
Biomydrin (P) 147
Bioral (P+▲) 16
BIPERIDEN 176
BISACODYL 30, 33
Bisacodyl (F) (P+▲) 30
   suppositories (F) (P+▲) 33
Bislumina (P+▲) 20
Bismag tablets and powder (▲)
   20
Bismodyne (P+▲) 35
BISMUTH 35
Bismuth subgallate compound
   suppository (F) (P+▲) 35
Bisodol tablets (P+▲) 20
Bisolvomycin (P) 63
Bisolvon (P) 52
BITOSCANATE 107
Bitoscanate BP (P+▲) 107
Bleph-10 liquifilm (P) 137
Bocasan (P+▲) 15
Bolvidon (P) 161, 162
Bonamint (▲) 30
Bonjela (P+▲) 17
Boots covering cream (▲) 87
Bradosol (P+▲) 152
BRAN 31
Bravisol (P+▲) 91
Brentan cream (P) 84
Breoprin (P+▲) 178
Brevinor (P) 112
Bricanyl (P) 41
Brocadopa (P) 175
Brolene (P+▲) 137
BROMAZEPAM 154
BROMELAINS AND CHYMOTRYPSIN
   131
BROMOCRIPTINE 99, 104, 175
BROMPHENIRAMINE 148
Bronchilator (P) 40
Bronchodil (P) 41
Bronchotone (P) 50
Bronhipax (▲) 43
Brontina (P) 44

Brontisol (P) 44
Brooklax (▲) 30
Brovon (P+▲) 42
Broxil (P) 60
Brufen (P) 126
Brulidine cream (P+▲) 81
BUCLIZINE (WITH NICOTINIC ACID)
   135
BUPRENORPHINE 182
Buscopan (P) 23
Butacote (P) 127
Butazolidin (P) 127
Butazolidin Alka (P) 127
Butazone (P) 127
BUTOBARBITONE 158
Butobarbitone (F) (P) 158
BUTORPHANOL 182
BUTRIPTYLINE 160, 162

Cafadol (P+▲) 190
Cafergot (P) 187–8
Caladryl (P+▲) 88
Calamine and Coal Tar (F)
   (P+▲) 95–6
Calamine products (F) (P+▲)
   88
Calcium carbonate powder
   compound (F) (P+▲) 20
CALCIUM SULPHALOXATE 64, 65
Califig (▲) 30
Callusolve (P+▲) 94
Calmurid (P+▲) 96
Calmurid HC (P) 96
Calpol (P+▲) 178
Calsalettes (P) 34
Calthor (P) 60
C.A.M. (P+▲) 42
Camcolit 250 and 400 (P) 167
Canesten cream (P+▲) 68–9,
   84
   duopack (P) 68–9
   powder (P) 84
   spray (P+▲) 84
Cantil (P) 24
Cantil with phenobarbitone (P)
   25
Capastat (P) 67
Capitol (P+▲) 79
Caprin (P+▲) 178
CARBAMAZEPINE 171, 189, 194
Carbellon (P+▲) 23
CARBENOXOLONE 16, 18, 21–2
CARBIMAZOLE 74
Carbo-Dome (P+▲) 95–6
CARBOXYMETHYLCELLULOSE 16
Cardophylin (P+▲) 45
CARFECILLIN 59
Carisoma Co (P) 190
Carter's Little Liver Pills (P) 34
CASCARA 30
Cascara tablets (F) (P+▲) 30
CASTER OIL 30
Caster Oil (F) (P+▲) 30
Caved-S (P+▲) 22
CEFACLOR 61
Celevac (P+▲) 27, 31, 54
Cellucon (P+▲) 27, 31, 55
CEPHALEXIN 61
Cephalexin (F) (P) 61
CEPHRADINE 61
Ceporex (P) 61
CERATONIA 27
Cerumol (P+▲) 144
Cervical cap (P+▲) 111

Cetavlex (P+▲) 79
Cetavlon (P+▲) 77
Cetiprin (P) 189
CETRIMIDE 77–8, 79
Cetrimide cream (F) (P+▲) 79
CETYLPYRIDINIUM 151
C-Film (P+▲) 110
CHALK AND KAOLIN PREPARATIONS 26
Chemocycline (P) 62
Chloractil (P) 168
CHLORAL HYDRATE 157
Chloral mixture (F) (P) 157
CHLORAMPHENICOL 63, 137, 145, 194
Chloramphenicol (F) (P) 137
ear drops (F) (P) 145
Chloraseptic (P+▲) 152
CHLORDIAZEPOXIDE 154, 194
CHLORHEXIDINE 79–80, 151
CHLORHEXIDINE GLUCONATE 15
CHLORINATED LIME 80
Chlorinated lime solution (P+▲) 80
CHLORMETHIAZOLE 157
CHLORMEZANONE 154
Chloromycetin (P) 137, 145
Chloromycetin Hydrocortisone (P) 139
CHLOROQUINE 128–9
CHLOROXYLENOL 80
Chloroxylenol solution (P+▲) 80
CHLORPHENESIN 83–4
Chlorphenesin cream and powder (F) (P+▲) 83–4
CHLORPHENIRAMINE 149
CHLORPROMAZINE 134, 168, 169
Chlorpromazine (F) (P) 168
CHLORPROTHIXENE 168, 169
CHLORTETRACYCLINE 62, 137
Choledyl (P+▲) 45
CHOLESTYRAMINE 29, 194, 195
CHOLINE AND CETALKONIUM 17
Chymoral (P) 131
CICLACILLIN 60
Cidomycin (P) 82
CIMETIDINE 21, 22
CINNARIZINE 133
Claradin (P+▲) 178
Clean & Clear (▲) 93
Clearasil (▲) 90
Clearine Eye-Drops (▲) 140
CLEMASTINE 149
CLINDAMYCIN SODIUM FUSIDATE 63
Clinoril (P) 126
CLIOQUINOL 145
CLIOQUINOL AND VITAMIN C 17
CLOBAZAM 155
CLOBETASOL 97
CLOBETASONE 97, 138
Clobetasone cream and ointment (F) (P) 97
Clomid (P) 99, 100
CLOMIPHENE CITRATE 99, 100
CLOMIPRAMINE 160, 162
CLOMOCYCLINE 62
CLONAZEPAM 171, 173
CLONIDINE 103, 185
CLOPENTHIXOL 168, 169
Clopixol (P) 168
CLORAZEPATE 155

CLOTRIMAZOLE 68–9, 84
CLOXACILLIN 60
COAL TAR 78, 95–6
Coal Tar and Salicylic ointment (F) (P+▲) 95–6
Coal Tar paste and paint (F) (P+▲) 95
Cobadex (P) 96
Codanin (▲) 190
CODEINE 178, 179
CODEINE AND MORPHINE/OPIUM PREPARATIONS 26–7
Codeine and Paracetamol (P+▲) 190
Codeine Linctus (F) (P+▲) 51
Codeine phosphate (F) (P) 26, 178
Codelcortone (P) 27, 47
Codelsol (P) 27
Codis Dispersible tablets (▲) 190
Cod Liver Oil (F) (▲) 131
Codural (▲) 190
Co-Ferol tablets (P) 119
Cogene (▲) 190
Cogentin (P) 176
Colchicine (P) 129
Coldrex tablets (▲) 150
Colifoam (P) 35
Colofac (P) 23
Cologel (P+▲) 27, 31
Coltapaste (P+▲) 95–6
Compound W (P+▲) 94
Concordin (P) 161, 163
Conova 30 (P) 112
Contac 400 Capsules (▲) 150
Copholco (P+▲) 52
Corlan (P) 16
Correctol (▲) 32
Corsodyl (P+▲) 15, 151
Cortacream (P) 96
Cortenema (P) 35
Corticaid (P) 139
Cosalgesic (▲) 190
Cosylan (P+▲) 51
CO-TRIMOXAZOLE 64, 65, 99, 194, 195
Co-trimoxazole tablets and mixtures (F) (P) 64
Covermark (▲) 87
Covonia (▲) 51
Cremalgex (P+▲) 124
Cremalgin (P+▲) 124
Cremathurm (P+▲) 124
CROMOGLYCATE 147
CROTAMITON 88–9
Crunch and Slim (P) 57
Crystapen G (P) 59
Crystapen V (P) 60
Cupal Wart Solvent (P) 94
Cuprimine (P) 128
Cutisan (▲) 83
Cyclimorph (P) 183
CYCLIZINE 133
CYCLOBARBITONE 159
Cyclobarbitone (F) (P) 159
Cyclo-Progynova (P) 102
CYPROHEPTADINE 149
CYPROTERONE 104

Dactil (P) 24
Daktarin
cream (P+▲) 84
oral gel (P+▲) 68, 69–70, 151

tablets (P+▲) 68, 69–70
Dalmane (P) 157
Daneral SA (P+▲) 149
DANTHRON 30
Daranide (P) 141
Dartalan (P) 168
Davenol (P+▲) 52
Day Nurse (▲) 150
DDD Lotion (▲) 90
Deanase DC (P) 131
Decadron (P) 47
Decortisyl (P) 47
Deep Heat (▲) 124, 125
Delfen (P+▲) 110
Delimon (P) 190
Deltacortone (P) 47
Deltacortril enteric (P) 27, 47
Delta-Phoricol (P) 27, 47
Deltastab (P) 27, 47
DEMECARIUM 142
DEMECLOCYCLINE 62
Dendrid (P) 137, 138
Depixol (P) 168
Dequadin (P+▲) 151
DEQUALINIUM 151
Dermaclean (▲) 90
Dermidex (▲) 88
Dermogesic (P+▲) 88
Dermonistat (P+▲) 84
Dermovate (P) 97
Deseril (P) 185–6
DESIPRAMINE 161, 162
Deteclo (P) 62
Dettol (▲) 80
Mouthwash (▲) 151
Dexacortisyl (P) 47
DEXAMETHASONE 47, 138
Dexa-Rhinaspray (P) 147
Dexedrine (P) 55
DEXTROMORAMIDE 182
DEXTROPROPOXYPHENE 178, 179
DEXTROPROPOXYPHENE/PARA-CETAMOL 178
DEXTROSE AND SODIUM CHLORIDE 27
DF 118 (P) 178
Diamorphine and cocaine elixir (Brompton cocktail) (P) 185
Diamorphine, cocaine and chlor-promazine elixir (P) 185
Diamorphine Linctus (F) (P) 51
Diamox (P) 141
Diamox Sustets (P) 141
Diatuss (P+▲) 51
DIAZEPAM 155, 194
Diazepam (F) (P) 155
DIBROMOPROPAMIDINE 81, 137
DICHLORALPHENAZONE 157
DICHLORPHENAMIDE 141
DICLOFENAC 126
Diconal (P) 182
DICYCLOMINE 24
Dienoestrol cream (P) 101
tablets (P) 101
DIETHYLPROPION 55
Difflam (P+▲) 124
Oral Rinse (P+▲) 151
DIFLUCORTOLONE 97
DIFLUNISAL 126, 178, 179, 194
Dihydergot (P) 188
DIHYDROCODEINE 178, 179–80
Dihydrocodeine and Para-cetamol (P+▲) 190
DI-ISO PRODUCT 110

Dijex (P+▲) 20
Diloran (P+▲) 20
DIMENHYDRINATE 133
DIMETHICONE 19, 20, 87
DIMETHICONE AND PANCREATIN
20
Dimethicone cream (F) (P+▲)
87
DIMETHINDENE 149
DIMETHOTHIAZINE 149
Dimotane (P+▲) 148
Expectorant (P+▲) 50
LA (P+▲) 148
Dimotapp (and Dimotapp LA
and P) (P+▲) 148
Dimyril Linctus (P) 52
Dioctyl-Medo (P+▲) 32, 33
Dioderm (P) 96
Dioralyte (P+▲) 27, 133
Diovol (P+▲) 20
DIPHENHYDRAMINE 133, 149
DIPHENOXYLATE IOPERAMIDE 27
DIPHENYLPYRALINE 149
DIPIPANONE 182
Disadine (P+▲) 81
Disalcid (P) 178
Disipal (P) 176
Disphex (▲) 81
Distaclor (P) 61
Distalgesic (P) 178, 190
Soluble (P) 190
Distamine (P) 128
Distaquaine VK (P) 60
Dithranol ointment and paste (F)
(P+▲) 96
DITHRANOL PREPARATIONS 95, 96
Dithrocream (P+▲) 96
Dithrolan (P+▲) 96
Dixarit (P) 103, 185
Doan's Backache Pills (▲) 191
DOCUSATE 33
DOCUSATE SODIUM 32
Do Do asthma pill (▲) 43
Dolasan (Lilly) (P) 191
Dolobid (P) 178
Doloxene (P) 178
Doloxene Compound (P) 191
Dome-Acne products (P+▲)
90
Dome-Cort (P) 96
Domical (P) 160, 161
DOMIPHEN BROMIDE 152
Dorbanex (P+▲) 30
Doriden (P) 159
DOTHIEPIN 161, 162
DOXEPIN 161, 162
DOXYCYCLINE 62, 195
Dramamine (P+▲) 133
Drapolene (P+▲) 79
Dristan Nasal Mist (▲) 147
Dristan tablets (▲) 150
Droleptan (P) 168
Dromoran (P) 182–3
DROPERIDOL 168, 169
Droxalin (P+▲) 20
Dubam (P+▲) 125
Dulcodos (F) (P+▲) 30
Dulcolax (F) (P+▲) 30
suppository (P+▲) 33
Dumas vault device (P+▲)
111
Duofilm (P+▲) 94
Duogastrone (P) 22
Duphalac (P+▲) 33

Duracreme (P+▲) 110
Duragel (P+▲) 110
Duromine (P) 56
Duromorph (P) 183
Durophet (▲) 55
Dust barrier cream (F) (P+▲)
87

Ebufac (P) 126
ECONAZOLE 68, 69, 84
Econazole nitrate cream (F) (P)
84
Economycin (P) 62
Ecostatin (P) 68, 69, 84
ECOTHIOPATE 142
Efcortelan (P) 96
Elamol (P) 165, 166
Elavil (P) 160, 161
Ellimans Embrocation (F) (▲)
124
Eltroxin (P) 73–4
Eludril (P+▲) 151
EMEPRONIUM 189
Emeside (P) 173
Emko (P+▲) 110
Emulsifying ointment (F)
(P+▲) 77
Enteromide (P) 64, 65
E.P. Tablets (▲) 191
Epanutin (P) 174
Epanutin and Phenobarbitone
Capsules (P) 174
EPHEDRINE 42, 43, 147, 194
Ephedrine hydrochloride
elixir (F) (P) 42
tablets (F) (P) 42
Ephedrine nasal drops (F) (P)
147
Epifrin (P) 142
Epilim (P) 172, 173
Eppy (P+▲) 142
Epsom Salts (P+▲) 33
Equagesic (P) 191
Equanil (P) 156
Equivert (P) 135
ERGOTAMINE 187–8
Erycen (P) 63
Erythrocin (P) 63
Erythromid (P) 63
ERYTHROMYCIN 63
Erythroped (P) 63
Eskamel (P+▲) 90–1
Eskornade (P+▲) 148
ETAMIPHYLLINE 45
Ethinyloestradiol tablets (P) 101
ETHOSUXIMIDE 173
Ethosuximide (F) (P) 173
ETHOTOIN 171
Etophylate (P+▲) 45
Eugynon (30 and 50) (P) 112
Euhypnos (P) 158
Eumovate (P) 97
Eumovate-N (P) 139
Eumovete (P) 138
Eumydrin (P) 44
Eurax ointment and lotion
(P+▲) 88–9
Eusol (P) 80
Evacalm (P) 155
Evadyne (P) 160, 162
Evidorm (P) 159
Ex-Lax (▲) 30
Exolan (P+▲) 96
Expansyl (P) 43

Exterol (P+▲) 144
Extil Compound (P+▲) 52
Eye Dew Eye-Drops (▲) 140

Fabahistin (P+▲) 149
Famel Expectorant (▲) 50
Famel Linctus (▲) 51
Famel Original (▲) 51
FEAC tablets (P+▲) 120
Fe-Cap capsule (P+▲) 118
Fe-Cap C capsules (P+▲) 120
Fe-Cap Folic Capsules (P) 119
Fefol Spansules (P) 119
Fefol-Vit Spansules (P) 120
Feldene (P) 126
Femerital (P+▲) 191
Feminax (▲) 191
Femulen (P) 115
FENBUFEN 126
FENCLOFENAC 126
FENFLURAMINE 55–6
FENOPROFEN 126, 178, 180
Fenopron (P) 178
Fenostil Retard (P+▲) 149
FENOTEROL 39–40
Fenox (P+▲) 147
Fentazin (P) 168
Feospan capsule (P+▲) 119
FEPRAZONE 126
Feravol-F tablets (P) 119
Feravol-G syrup (▲) 120
Feravol-G tablets (▲) 120
Feravol syrup (▲) 120
Feravol tablets (▲) 120
Ferfolic SV tablets (P) 120
Ferfolic tablets (P) 120
Fergluvite tablets (P+▲) 121
Fergon tablet (P+▲) 118
Ferraplex B tablets (P+▲) 121
Ferrlecit 100 tablets (P+▲)
121
Ferrocap capsules (P+▲) 121
Ferrocap-F 350 capsules (P)
119
Ferrocontin Continus tablets
(P+▲) 118
Ferrocontin F Continus tablets
(P) 120
Ferrograd C tablets (P+▲) 121
Ferro-Gradumet tablet (P+▲)
119
Ferromyn B elixir and tablets
(P+▲) 121
Ferromyn elixir (5 ml) (P+▲)
119
Ferromyn S Folic tablets (P) 121
Ferromyn S tablets (P) 121
Ferromyn tablet (P+▲) 119
FERROUS FUMARATE REMEDIES
118
Ferrous fumarate tablet (P+▲)
118
FERROUS GLUCONATE REMEDIES
118
Ferrous gluconate tablet (P+▲)
118
FERROUS GLYCINE REMEDIES 118
FERROUS SUCCINATE REMEDIES
119
Ferrous succinate tablet (P+▲)
119
Ferrous sulphate mixture (5 ml)
(P+▲) 119
FERROUS SULPHATE REMEDIES 119

Ferrous sulphate tablet (P+▲) 119
Compound (P+▲) 120
Fersaday tablet (P+▲) 118
Fersamal syrup (5 cc) (P+▲) 118
Fersamel tablet (P+▲) 118
Fesovit Spansules (P+▲) 121
FIG 30
Flagyl (P) 151
FLAVOXATE 190
Flenac (P) 126
Fletcher's Beogex Phosphate Enema (P+▲) 33
Fletcher's Magnesium sulphate enema (P+▲) 33
Fletcher's Oil enema (P+▲) 33
Flosint (P) 126
Floxapen (P) 60
Fluanxol (P) 165, 166
FLUCLOXACILLIN 60
FLUCLOXACILLIN + AMPICILLIN 60
FLUCOROLONE 97
FLUFENAMIC ACID 126, 178, 180
FLUOCINOLONE 97
FLUOCINONIDE 97
FLUOCORTOLONE 97
FLUOROMETHOLONE 138
FLUPENTHIXOL 165, 166, 168, 169
FLUPHENAZINE 168, 169
FLURANDRENOLONE 96
FLURAZEPAM 157
FLURBIPROFEN 126
FML Liquifilm (P) 138
Folex-350 tablets (P) 120
Folicin tablets (P) 121
Folvron tablets (P) 120
Forceval capsules (P+▲) 121
FORMALDEHYDE 94
Formulary sulphur (F) (P+▲) 91
Fortagesic (P) 191
Fortral (P) 178
FRAMYCETIN 63, 81–2, 137, 145
FRAMYCETIN WITH STEROID 145
Framycort (P) 139, 145
Framygen (P) 81, 137, 145
Franol (P) 43
Franol Expectorant (P+▲) 50
Franolyn Expectorant (▲) 50
Frisium (P) 155
Froben (P) 126
Fucidin (P) 63, 82
Fulcin (P) 68, 69
Fungilin (P) 68, 83, 151
FUSAFUNGINE 152
FUSIDIC ACID 82
Furacin (P) 82
Fybogel (P+▲) 31
Fybranta (P+▲) 31
Fynnon Calcium Asprin (▲) 178

Galenomycin (P) 62
Galfer capsule (P+▲) 118
Galfer FA capsules (P) 120
Galloways Bronchial Expectorant (▲) 50
Galloways Cough Syrup (▲) 51
Ganda (P) 142
Gantrisin (P) 64, 66

Garoin (P) 174
Gastalar (P+▲) 20
Gastrocote (P+▲) 18
Gastrovite tablets (P+▲) 121
Gatinar (P+▲) 33
Gaviscon (P+▲) 18
Gelusil (P+▲) 20
Genasprin (▲) 178
Genexol (P+▲) 110
GENTAMICIN 63, 82, 137, 145
GENTAMICIN WITH HYDROCORTISONE 145
Genticin (P) 82, 137, 145
Gentisone HC (P) 145
Germolene (▲) 93
Germoloids (P+▲) 35
Gevral capsules (P+▲) 121
Glacial acetic acid (F) (P+▲) 94
Glaubers Salts (P+▲) 33
GLUTARALDEHYDE 94, 95
Glutarol (P+▲) 94, 95
GLUTETHIMIDE 159
GLYCEROL 33
Glycerol (F) (P+▲) 144
suppositories (P+▲) 33
GLYCOPYRRONIUM 24
Glykola Elixir (P+▲) 121
Graneodin (P) 137
Gravol (P+▲) 133
GRISEOFULVIN 68, 69, 195
Griseofulvin (F) (P) 68, 69
Grisovin (P) 68, 69
GUANETHIDINE REMEDIES 142
Gyno-Daktarin (P) 68, 69–70
Gyno-Pevaryl (P) 68, 69
Gynovlar 21 (P) 112

Haelan (P) 96
Halciderm (P) 97
HALCINONIDE 97
Halcort (P) 97
Haldol (P) 168
HALOPERIDOL 168, 169, 176
Haloperidol (P) 168
HALQUINOL WITH STEROID 145
HAMAMELIS 35
Hamamelis and zinc suppository (F) (P+▲) 35
Hamamelis suppository (F) (P+▲) 35
Harmogen (P) 102
Havapen (P) 60
Haymine (P+▲) 149
Hayphryn (P+▲) 147
Hedex (P+▲) 178
Hedex Seltzer (▲) 191
Heminevrin (P) 157
Hepacort Plus (P) 36
HEPTABARBITONE 159
Hermesetas (▲) 57
Herpid (P) 70, 71
HEXACHLOROPHANE 80
Hexachlorophane dusting powder (P+▲) 80
HEXETIDINE 15–16, 152
Hibiscrub (P+▲) 79
Hibisol (P+▲) 79
Hibitane (P+▲) 79
Hills Bronchial Balsam (▲) 51
Hills Junior Balsam (▲) 51
Hioxyl (P+▲) 80
Histalix (P+▲) 148
Histryl (P+▲) 149

Hormofemin cream (P) 101
Hormonin (P) 101
HPD (▲) 57
HYDROCORTISONE 16, 35, 47, 96
Hydrocortisone (F) (P) 96
HYDROCORTISONE ACETATE 96
Hydrocortisone acetate ointment (F) (P) 96
HYDROCORTISONE BUTYRATE 97
Hydrocortisone suppositories (F) (P) 35
Hydrocortistab (P) 47, 96
Hydrocortisyl (P) 96
Hydrocortone (P) 47, 96
HYDROGEN PEROXIDE 80
Hydrogen Peroxide solution (P+▲) 80
HYDROTALCITE 20
HYDROTALCITE AND DIMETHICONE 20
Hydrous wool fat (F) (P+▲) 86
HYDROXYZINE 155
HYOSCINE 132
Hyoscine tablets (F) (P) 132
HYOSCYAMINE 23
Hypon (P+▲) 191
HYPROMELLOSE EYE DROPS 143

Iberet 500 tabets (P+▲) 121
Iberol Filmtabs (P+▲) 121
IBUPROFEN 126
Ibuprofen tablets (P) 126
Icipen (P) 60
Icthaband (P+▲) 96
ICHTHAMMOL 95, 96
Ichthammol bandage and ointment (F) (P+▲) 96
Ichthopaste (P+▲) 96
Idocid (P) 127
Idocid R (P) 127
Idoxene (P) 137, 138
IDOXURIDINE 70, 71, 137, 138
Idoxuridine (F) (P) 137, 138
Iliadin (P+▲) 147
Ilosone (P) 63
Ilotycin (P) 63
Imbrilon (P) 127
IMIPRAMINE 161, 162
Imodium (P) 27
Imperacin (P) 62
Inderal and Inderal LA (P) 156–7
INDOMETHACIN 127, 195
Indomethacin (F) (P) 127, 129
INDOPROFEN 126
Inolaxine (P+▲) 31
Intal and Intal Co (P) 49
Integrin (P) 168
Intralgin (P+▲)77) 124
IODINE 74
Ionamin (P) 56
Ionax scrub (P+▲) 91–2
Ionil T (P+▲) 78
Ipecacuanha and Morphine Mixture (F) (P+▲) 50
IPRATROPIUM 44
IPRINDOLE 161, 162
IPRONIAZID 165
Irofol Filmtabs (P) 121
Iron Jelloids (▲) 121
Ironorm Capsules (P) 121
Ironorm Tonic with Iron (P) 122
Iron Plan (▲) 122
Ismelin (P) 142

Iso-Autohaler (P) 42
Iso-Brovon inhaler (P) 42
ISOETHARINE 40
Isoforte (P) 42
Isogel (P+▲) 27, 31
Isopto Alkaline (P+▲) 143
Isopto cetamide (P) 137
Isopto Epinal (P+▲) 142
Isopto Plain (P+▲) 143
Isopto-Carpine (P) 142
ISOPRENALINE 42-3
Isoprenaline tablets (F) (P) 42
ISPAGHULA 27
ISPAGHULA HUSK 31

Joyrides (▲) 132
Juno Juniper Salts (P) 33

Kaolin and morphine (F) (P+▲)
  26
  mixture (P+▲) 26
Kaolin/soap skin conditioning
  cream (F) (P+▲) 87
Kaopectate (F) (P+▲) 26
Karvol Inhalant Capsules (▲)
  148
Kaylene-Ol and liquid paraffin
  mixture (F) (P+▲) 32
Kaylene-OL with phenol-
  phthalein (P+▲) 30
Kelferon tablet (P+▲) 118
Keflex (P) 61
Kelfizine W (P) 64, 65
Kelfolate tablets (P) 120
Kemadrin (P) 176
Kerecid (P) 137, 138
Kest (P+▲) 33
KETAZOLAM 155-6
KETOCONAZOLE 68, 69
KETOPROFEN 126
Ketoprofen capsules and sup-
  pository (P) 126
Klyx (P+▲) 33
Kolanticon (P+▲) 24
Kolantyl (P+▲) 24
Kwells (▲) 132

Laboprin (P+▲) 178
Labosept (P+▲) 151
Lac bismuth (P+▲) 20
LACTULOSE 33
Lactulose elixir (F) (P+▲) 33
Lanacane (▲) 88
Largactil (P) 134, 168
Larodopa (P) 175
Lasonil (P+▲) 35
Ledercort (P) 47, 97
Lederfen (P) 126
Lederkyn (P) 64, 65
Ledermycin (P) 62
Lemsip sachets (▲) 150
Lenium shampoo (P+▲) 78
Lentizol (P) 160, 161
Lergoban (P+▲) 149
Lessen (▲) 57
Levius (P+▲) 178
LEVODOPA 175, 194
Levodopa (F) (P) 175
LEVORPHANOL 182-3
Lexotan (P) 154
Libraxin (P) 25
Librium, Tropium and Chlor-
  diazepoxide preparation (F)
  (P) 154

Limmits (▲) 57
LINCTUS ELIXIR REMEDIES 52
Lingraine (P) 188
LIOTHYRONINE SODIUM 74
Liqufruta (▲) 51
LIQUID PARAFFIN 32
Liquid Paraffin with magnesium
  hydroxide (F) (P+▲) 32
Liquid Paraffin with phenolph-
  thalein (F) (P+▲) 31, 32
Liquifilm Tears (P+▲) 143
LIQUORICE 22
Liskonum (P) 167
Listerine Antiseptic (▲) 151
LITHIUM CARBONATE 167
Lloyd's cream (▲) 124
Lobak (P) 191
Locabiotal (P) 152
Locan (▲) 88
Locoid (P) 97
Locorten-Vioform (P) 145
Loestrin 20 (P) 112
Logynon and Logynon ED (P)
  113
Lomotil (P) 27
Lomusol (P+▲) 147
LORAZEPAM 156
Lotussin (P+▲) 52
Ludiomil (P) 161, 162
Luminal (P) 171-2
LYMECYCLINE 62

Maalox and Maalox plus (P+▲)
  20
Maclean's tablets and powder
  (P+▲) 20
Madopar (P) 175
Madribon (P) 64, 65
MAFENIDE 137
Magnapen (P) 60
Magnesia (P) 33
Magnesium carbonate powder
  compound (F) (P+▲) 20
Magnesium carbonate tablets
  compound (F) (P+▲) 20
MAGNESIUM COMPOUNDS 33
MAGNESIUM HYDROXIDE 19
MAGNESIUM PREPARATIONS 19
Magnesium sulphate and
  hydroxide mixtures (P+▲)
  19
Magnesium trisilicate (F) (P+▲
  19
  and belladonna (F) (P+▲)
  23
Malarivon (P) 128
M & B antiseptic cream (P+▲)
  82
M & B 693 (P) 64
MAPROTILINE 161, 162
Marsilid (P) 165
Marvelon (P) 113
Marzine (P+▲) 133
Maxidex (P) 138
Maxitrol (P) 139
Maxolon (P) 24, 134
MAZINDOL 56
MEBENDAZOLE 106
MEBEVERINE 23
MEBHYDROLIN 149
MECLOZINE 133
MEDAZEPAM 156
Medihaler-Duo (P) 42
Medihaler-Epi (P) 42

Medihaler-Iso (P) 42
Medijel (P+▲) 17
Medilave (P+▲) 16
Medocodene (P) 191
Medomin (P) 159
Medrone (P) 47
Medrone Acne Lotion (P) 92
MEFANAMIC ACID 126, 178, 180
Megaclor (P) 62
Melleril (P) 104, 168
Menophase (P) 102
Mentholatum Balm (▲) 148
MEPACRINE 108
Mepacrine Tablets BP (P+▲)
  108
MEPENZOLATE 24
Meprate (P) 156
MEPROBAMATE 156
Meprobamate (F) (P) 156
MEPTAZINOL 183
Meptid (P) 183
MEPYRAMINE 149
MEQUITAZINE 149
Meralen (P) 178
Merbentyl (P+▲) 24
Mercuric Oxide (F) (▲) 140
Merital (P) 161, 163
Merocets (P+▲) 151
MESTEROLONE 99
Metamucil (P+▲) 31
METAZOLINE DERIVATIVES 147
METHACYCLINE 62
Methadone (P) 183
METHIXENE 176
METHOXYPHENAMINE 43
Methrazone (P) 126
METHYLCELLULOSE 27, 31
Methylcellulose granules (F)
  (P+▲) 27, 31
METHYLPHENOBARBITONE 171
METHYLPREDNISOLONE 47
Methyl Salicylate Liniment (F)
  (P+▲) 123
Methyl Salicylate Ointment (F)
  (P+▲) 124
METHYLTESTOSTERONE 99
METHYPRYLONE 159
METHYSERGIDE 185-6
Metilar (P) 47
METOCLOPRAMIDE 24-5, 134,
  194
Metosyn (P) 97
METRONIDAZOLE 151, 195
MEXENONE 86
Mexenone cream (F) (P+▲) 86
MIANSERIN 161, 162
MICONAZOLE 68, 69-70, 84,
  151
Miconazole (F) (P) 68, 69-70
Miconazole nitrate (F) (P) 84
Micralax (P+▲) 33
Microgynon 30 (P) 113
Micronor (P) 115
Microval (P) 115
Midrid (P) 187
Migraleve (P) 186
Migravess (P) 186-7
Migril (P) 188
Milk of Magnesia (▲) 19
Millophyline (P) 45
Milonorm (P) 156
Milpar (P+▲) 32
Miltown (P) 156
Minadex syrup (▲) 122

Minilyn (P) 113
Minims chloramphenicol (P) 137
Minims neomycin sulphate (P) 137
Minims Pilocarpine Nitrate (P) 142
Minims sulphacetamide (P) 137
Minocin (P) 62
MINOCYCLINE 62
Minovlar and Minovlar ED (P) 113
Mintezol (P) 106, 108
Mixogen (P) 103
Mobilan (P) 127
Moditen (P) 168
Mogadon (P) 158
Molcer (P+▲) 144
Molipaxin (P) 161, 163, 165, 166
Monistat (P+▲) 68, 69–70
Monotheamin (P+▲) 45
Monphytal (P+▲) 85
Moorlands tablets (P+▲) 20
Morhulin (P+▲) 86
MORPHINE 183
Morphine and cocaine elixir (P) 185
Morphine, cocaine and chlorpromazine elixir (P) 185
Morphine injection and suppository (F) (P) 183
Morsep (P+▲) 79
Movelat (P) 124
MST Continus (P) 183
Mucodyne (P) 52
Mucolex (P) 52
MUCOLYTIC REMEDIES 52
Mucron Children's Liquid (▲) 150
Mucron tablets (▲) 150
Murine Eye-Drops (▲) 140
Myambutol (P) 67
Myciguent (P) 82, 137
Mycil (P+▲) 83–4
Mycota (P+▲) 85
Myolgin Dispersible Tablets (P+▲) 191
Mysoline (P) 172
Mysoline and Phenytoin tablets 174
Mysteclin (P) 63

Nacton (P) 24
Nalcrom (P) 28
NAPROXEN 126, 129, 178, 180, 194
Naproxen (F) (P) 129
Napsalgesic (P) 191
Nardil (P) 164–5
Narphen (P) 184
NATAMYCIN 68, 70, 84
Natrena (▲) 57
Natuderm (▲) 87
Naxogin (P+▲) 15
NEFOPAM 183–4
Nembutal (P) 159
Neo-Cortef (P) 139, 145
Neogest (P) 115
Neo-Medrone (P) 92
Neo-Mercazole (P) 74
NEOMYCIN 63, 81, 82, 196
Neomycin cream (F) (P) 82
NEOMYCIN/GRAMICIDIN 137, 138

NEOMYCIN WITH STEROID 145
Neophryn (P+▲) 147
Neosporin (P) 139
Nepenthe (P) 183
Nerisone (P) 97
Nestolyn (P+▲) 35
Neulactil (P) 168
Neurodol (▲) 191
Neurodyne (▲) 191
Neutradonna (P+▲) 23
Neutrolactis (P+▲) 20
NICLOSAMIDE 107–8
Niferex elixir (5 ml) (P+▲) 119
Niferex tablet (P+▲) 119
Night Nurse (▲) 150
Nilstim (P+▲) 55
NIMORAZOLE 15
Nitoman (P) 176
Nitrados (P) 158
NITRAZEPAM 158
Nitrazepam mixture (F) (P) 158
NITROFURAZONE 82
Nivaquine (P) 128
Nizoral (P) 68, 69
Nobrium (P) 156
Noctec and Chloral mixture (F) (P) 157
Noludar (P) 159
NOMIFENSINE 161, 163
NONOXINOL PRODUCTS 110
Noradran (P+▲) 42
Norflex (P) 176
Norgesic (P) 191
Norgeston (P) 115
Norgotin (P+▲) 146
Noriday (P) 115
Norimin (P) 113
Norinyl-1 (P) 113
Norlestrin (P) 113
Normacol (P+▲) 30
    Antispasmodic (P+▲) 31
    Special (P+▲) 31
    Standard (P+▲) 31
    Standard sugar-free (P+▲) 31
Normax (P+▲) 30
Normison (P) 158
NORTRIPTYLINE 161, 163
Norval (P) 161, 162
Nuelin and Nuelin SA (P+▲) 45
Nulacin (P+▲) 20
Numotac (P) 40
Nu-Seals Aspirin (P+▲) 178
Nylax (▲) 31
Nystan (P) 68, 70, 84–5, 151
NYSTATIN 68, 70, 84–5, 151
Nystavescent (P) 68, 70

Ocusert (P) 142
Ocusol (P) 137, 139
Oestradiol (F) (P) 101
Oestriol (F) (P) 101
Oilatum cream (P+▲) 77
Oilatum emollient (P+▲) 77
Oil-repellent barrier (F) (P+▲) 87
Oily cream (F) (P+▲) 86
Olbas Oil (▲) 148
Olive oil (F) (P+▲) 144
Omnopon and papaveretum injection (F) (P) 184
Onadox-118 (P) 191

Opas tablets and powder (P+▲) 20
Ophthalmadine (P) 137, 138
Opium tincture (F) (P) 183
Optabs Eye Lotion Solution Tablets (▲) 140
Opticrom (P) 140
Optimax and Optimax WV (P) 165, 166
Optimine (P+▲) 148
Optrex Drops (▲) 140
Optrex Eye Lotion (▲) 140
Optrex Eye Ointment (▲) 140
Orabase (P+▲) 16
Oradexon (P) 47
Oralcer (P+▲) 17
Oraldene (P+▲) 15, 152
Orap (P) 168
Oratrol (P) 141
Orbenin (P) 60
ORCIPRENALINE 43
Organidin (P+▲) 52
Orlest 21 (P) 113
ORPHENADRINE 176
Ortho-Creme (P+▲) 110
Ortho-Forms (P+▲) 110
Ortho-Gynol jelly (P+▲) 110
Ortho-Novin 1/50 (P) 113
Orthoxine (P+▲) 43
Orudis (P) 126
Oruvail (P) 126
Osmosin (P) 127
Ospolot (P) 172–3
Otopred (P) 145
Otoseptil (P) 146
Otosporin (P) 146
Ototrips (P) 146
Otrivine (P+▲) 147
Otrivine-Antistin (P+▲) 139
Ovestin (P) 101
Ovol (P) 24
Ovran and Ovran 30 (P) 113
Ovranette (P) 113
Ovulen 50 (P) 113
Ovysmen (P) 113
Owbridges Cough Syrup (▲) 51
OXATOMIDE 149
OXAZEPAM 156
Oxymycin (P) 62
OXYPERTINE 168, 169, 194
OXYPHENBUTAZONE 140
OXYTETRACYCLINE 62
Oxytetracycline (F) (P) 62
OXYTETRACYCLINE AND BROMHEXINE 63
OXYTETRACYCLINE, EPHEDRINE AND IPECACUANHA 63

Pacaps (P) 55
Pacitron (P) 165, 166
PADIMATE 86
Paedo-Sed (▲) 191
Palfium (P) 182
Pamergan AP (P) 184
Pamergan P100 (P) 184
Panadeine Co (P+▲) 191
Panadol (P+▲) 178
Panasorb (P+▲) 178
PANCREATIN 20
Panets (P+▲) 178
Panoxyl (P+▲) 91
PAPAVERETUM 184
Parabal (P) 171–2
PARACETAMOL 178, 180–1, 194

Paracetamol tablets and elixir (F) (P+▲) 178
Paracodol (P+▲) 191
Paradeine (▲) 191
Paraffin ointment (F) (P+▲) 86
Paraffin-type oil-repellent (F) (P+▲) 87
Paragesic (P+▲) 148
Parahypon (P+▲) 191
Parake (P+▲) 191
Paralgin (P+▲) 191
Paramax (P) 187
PARAMETHASONE 47
Paramol-118 (P) 191
Parazolidin (P) 191
Pardale (P+▲) 191
Parlodel (P) 100, 175
Parnate (P) 165
Paxidal (▲) 191
Paynocil (P+▲), 178
PECILOCIN 85
PECTIN 20
Peganone (P) 171
PENAMECILLIN 60
Penbritin (P) 59
Pendramine (P) 128
Penetrol Inhalant (▲) 148
PENICILLAMINE 128, 195
Penidural (P) 59
PENTAZOCINE 178, 181
PENTOBARBITONE 159
Pentovis (P) 102
Pentrexyl (P) 59
Peptard (P) 23
Peralvex (P+▲) 17
Periactin (P+▲) 149
PERICYAZINE 168, 169
Peroidin (P) 74-5
PERPHENAZINE 168, 169
Persomnia (P) 158
Pertofran (P) 161, 162
PETHIDINE 184, 194
Pethidine tablets and injections (F) (P) 184
Pethilorfan (P) 184
Petrolagar No. 1 (P+▲) 32
Petrolagar No. 2 (P+▲) 30
Pevaryl (P) 68, 69, 84
Phanodorm (P) 159
Pharmidone (P+▲) 191
Phasal (P) 167
Phazyme (P+▲) 20
PHENAZOCINE 184
PHENAZOPYRIDINE 189
PHENELZINE 164-5
Phenergan (P+▲) 133, 149, 158
Phenergan Compound Expectorant (P+▲) 50
PHENETHICILLIN 60
PHENINDAMINE 149
PHENIRAMINE 149
PHENOBARBITONE 43, 171-2, 194, 195
Phenobarbitone (F) (P) 159, 171-2
Phenobarbitone Spansule (P) 171-2
PHENOL 152
PHENOLPHTHALEIN 30-1
Phenolphthalein tablets (F) (P+▲) 31
PHENOXYMETHYLPENICILLIN (PENICILLIN V) 60

Phenoxymethylpenicillin (F) (P) 60, 196
Phensedyl Linctus (P+▲) 51
Phensic (▲) 192
PHENTERMINE 56
Phenylbutazone (F) (P) 127, 129, 194, 195, 196
PHENYLBUTAZONE AND OXY-PHENBUTAZONE 127-8
PHENYTOIN 172, 194, 195, 196
Phenytoin (F) (P) 172
Phillips Iron Tonic (▲) 122
pHiso-Ac (▲) 91
PHiso-Hex (P+▲) 80
PHiso-Med (P+▲) 80
Pholcodine Linctus (P+▲) 51
Pholcolix (P+▲) 51
Pholcomed (P+▲) 51
  Diabetic (P+▲) 51
  Expectorant Syrup (P+▲) 50
  Forte (P+▲) 51
  Forte Diabetic (P+▲) 51, 52
  Pastilles (P+▲) 51
PHOSPHATES 33
Phosphates enema A+B (F) (P+▲) 33
Phospholine Iodine (P) 142
PHTHALYSULPHATHIAZOLE 64, 65
Phyllocontin (P+▲) 45
Phyllosan (▲) 122
Physeptone (P) 183
Physostigmine (F) (P) 142
Physostigmine and Pilocarpine drops (F) (P) 142
PHYSOSTIGMINE AND PILOCARPINE REMEDIES 142
Pilocarpine (F) (P) 142
Pimafucin (P) 68, 70, 84
PIMOZIDE 168, 169
PIPENZOLATE 24
PIPERAZINE 105-6
Piperazine Elix (▲) 105
PIPERIDOLATE 24
Piptal (P) 24
Piptalin (P) 24
Piriton (P+▲) 149
PIROXICAM 126
PIVAMPICILLIN 60
PIZOTIFEN 186
Plaquenil (P) 128
Plesmet syrup (5 ml) (P+▲) 118
PODOPHYLLUM 93, 94
Podophyllum paint (F) (P+▲) 93, 94
POLDINE 24
Polyalk (P+▲) 20
  suspension and gel (P+▲) 20
Polycrol (P+▲) 20
POLYETHYLENE 91-2
Polyfax (P) 137, 139
POLYMIXIN B SULPHATE 137
POLYNOXYLIN 82, 151
POLYSACCHARIDE-IRON COMPLEX TABLETS 119
Polytar (P+▲) 78
Polytrim (P) 137
POLYVINYL ALCOHOL 143
Ponderax (P) 55
Pondocillin (P) 60
Ponoxylan (P+▲) 82
Ponstan (P) 178

Posalfilin (P+▲) 93, 94
POTASSIUM PERCHLORATE 74-5
Potter's Catarrh Pastilles (▲) 150
POVIDONE-IODINE 80-1, 152
Practo-Clyss (P+▲) 33
Precortisyl (P) 27, 47
Predenema (P) 35
Prednesol (P) 47
PREDNISOLONE 27, 35, 47, 128, 138, 145
Prednisolone tablets (F) (P) 27, 47
PREDNISONE 47
Prednisone (F) (P) 47
Predsol (P) 35, 138, 145
Predsol-N (P) 139, 145
Prefil (P+▲) 55
Pregaday tablets (P) 120
Pregavite Forte F tablets (P) 122
Pregfol capsules (P) 120
Premarin (P) 102
  cream (P) 101
Prempak (P) 102
Preparation H (P+▲) 35
Priadel (P) 167
Primalan (P) 149
PRIMIDONE 172, 194, 195
Primperan (P) 24
Pripsen (▲) 105
Pro-Actidil (P) 149
Pro-Banthine (P) 24
  with Dartalan (P) 25
PROBENECID 130, 194, 195, 196
PROCHLORPERAZINE 134-5
Proctofibe (P+▲) 31
Proctofoam HC (P) 36
Procol Capsules (▲) 150
PROCYCLIDINE 176
Proctosedyl (P) 36
Prodexin (P+▲) 20
Product Earwax (P+▲) 144
Progesic (P) 178
Progynova (P) 101
PROMAZINE 168, 169
PROMETHAZINE 133, 149, 158
Promethazine (F) (P) 158
Prominal (P) 171
Prondol (P) 161, 162
Propa PH (P+▲) 77, 79
Propaderm (P) 97
Propain (P+▲) 192
PROPAMIDINE 82
PROPANTHELINE 24
Propantheline tablets (F) (P) 24
PROPRANOLOL 156-7
Propranolol tablets (F) (P) 156-7
PROPYLTHIOURACIL 75
Propylthiouracil tablets (F) (P) 75
Prothiaden (P) 161, 162
PROTRIPTYLINE 161, 163
Pro-Viron (P) 99
PROXYPHYLLINE 45
PR Spray (P+▲) 125
Psoradrate (P) 96
Psoriderm (P+▲) 95-6
Pulmadil (P) 40
Pulmo Bailly (▲) 50
Pyorex (P+▲) 16, 151
Pyralvex (P+▲) 151
Pyridium (P+▲) 189
Pyrogastrone (▲) 18, 22

Questran (P) 29
QUINALBARBITONE 159
Quinoderm (P+▲) 91
    cream with hydrocortisone
    (P) 93

Rabro (P+▲) 22
Radian B aerosol (▲) 125
    Spirit Liniment (▲) 124
Radian Massage Cream (▲)
    125
Ralgex Balm (▲) 125
Ralgex Aerosol (▲) 125
Ralgex Stick (▲) 124
RANITIDINE 21
Rehidrat (P+▲) 27
Relaxit (P+▲) 33
Remnos (P) 158
Remotic (P) 145
Rendells (P+▲) 110
Rennies tablets (P+▲) 20
REPROTERAL 41
RESERPINE 104, 194
RESORCINOL 90-1
Resorcinol preparations (F)
    (P+▲) 91
Retcin (P) 63
Retin-A (P) 92
Rheumox (P) 125
Rhinamid (P) 147
RHUBARB 34
Rhubarb and soda mixture (F)
    (P+▲) 34
Rhubarb mixture compound (F)
    (P+▲) 34
Rifadin (P) 67
Rimactane (P) 67
Rimifon (P) 67
RIMITEROL 40
Rinstead Gel and Pastilles
    (P+▲) 17
Rinurel (P+▲) 148
Rinurel SA (P) 148
Rivotril (P) 171, 173
Robaxisal Forte (P) 192
Robinul (P) 24
Robitussin (P+▲) 52
Roccal (P+▲) 79
Rona-Slophyllin (P+▲) 45
Rondomycin (P) 62
Roter (P+▲) 20
Rotersept (P+▲) 80
Rybarvin (P+▲) 42
Rynacrom (P+▲) 147

SACCHARIN 57
SACCHARIN AND SUGAR COMBI-
    NATIONS 57
Safapryn and Safapryn Co
    (P+▲) 192
Salactol (P+▲) 94
SALBUTAMOL 40-1
Salazopyrin (P) 28
SALICYLIC ACID 90, 93
Salicylic acid and sulphur cream
    (F) (P+▲) 90
Salicylic Acid Collodion (F)
    (P+▲) 94
SALSALATE 178, 181
Salzone (P+▲) 178
Sancos (P+▲) 52
Sanomigran (P) 186
Saroten (P) 160, 161

Savlon (P+▲) 77
    cream (▲) 79
Saxin (▲) 57
Scheriproct (P) 36
Sealegs (P+▲) 133
Seconal (P) 159
Sedapam (P) 155
Sedonan (P+▲) 146
SELENIUM SULPHIDE 78-9
Selenium sulphide (F) (P) 78
Selsun shampoo (P+▲) 79
Senade (P+▲) 31
SENNA 31
Senokot (P+▲) 31
Septrin (P) 64, 65
Serc (P) 135
Sereen (▲) 132
Serenace (P) 168
Serenid-D (P) 156
Serenid Forte (P) 156
Setlers tablets (P+▲) 20
Seven seas bran (▲) 31
Sevilan (▲) 93
Sidros tablets (P+▲) 122
Silbe inhalant (P) 44
Silbephylline (P+▲) 45
Siloxyl and Siloxyl suspension
    (P+▲) 20
Simplene (P) 142
Sinemet (P) 175
Sine-Off tablets (▲) 150
Sinequan (P) 161, 162
Sintisone (P) 27, 47
Siopel (P+▲) 87
Skefron (P+▲) 125
Slender (▲) 57
    Bars (▲) 57
    Slim Soups (▲) 57
Slimgard (▲) 57
    5-Day Diet (▲) 57
Slim Line (▲) 56
Slim Plan (▲) 57
Sloan's Liniment (▲) 124
Slow-Fe Folic tablets (P) 120
Slow-Fe tablets (P+▲) 119
Sno-Phenicol (P) 137
Sno Pilo (P) 142
SOAP AND SPIRIT 79
Sodium Amytal (P) 158
SODIUM BICARBONATE 19
Sodium bicarbonate drops (F)
    (P+▲) 144
Sodium bicarbonate tablets (F)
    (P+▲) 19
SODIUM CROMOGLYCATE 28-9,
    49, 140
SODIUM IRON VEDETATE 119
SODIUM PERBORATE MONOHYDRATE
    AND HYDROGEN TARTRATE 15
SODIUM SALICYLATE 178, 181
Sodium salicylate mixture (F)
    (P+▲) 178
SODIUM SALTS 33
SODIUM VALPROATE 172, 173,
    194
Sofradex (P) 146
Soframycin (P) 137, 146, 147
Sofra-Tulle (P) 82
Soft soap (P+▲) 79
Solis (P) 155
Soliwax (P+▲) 144
Solpadeine (P+▲) 192
Solprin/Disprin (P+▲) 178
Somnite (P) 158

Soneryl (P) 158
Sovol (▲) 20
Sparine (P) 168
Spasmonal (P+▲) 23
Spectraban (P+▲) 86
Spirit soap (P+▲) 79
Spotaway (▲) 93
Sprilon (P+▲) 87
Squill Linctus Opiate (F) (P+▲)
    52
Stabillin VK (P) 60
Stadol (P) 182
Staycept (P+▲) 110
Stelabid (P) 25
Stelazine (P) 168
Stemetil (P) 134-5
STERCULIA 31
STEROID PREPARATIONS 95, 96-7,
    147
STEROID WITH ANTIBIOTICS 92-3
Ster-Zac powder (P+▲) 80
Stie-Lasan (P+▲) 96
Stilboestrol pessaries (P) 101
Streptotriad 64, 66
Sturgeron (P+▲) 133
Sucron (▲) 57
Sudafed (P+▲) 43, 148
Sudafed Co (P+▲) 148
Sudafed Expectorant (P+▲) 51
Suga Twin (▲) 57
SULFAMETOPYRAZINE 64, 65
Sulfapred (P) 139
Sulfomyl (P+▲) 137
SULINDAC 126
SULPHACETAMIDE 137
SULPHADIAZINE 64, 66
SULPHADIMETHOXINE 64, 65
SULPHADIMIDINE 64, 66
SULPHAFURAZOLE 64, 66
SULPHAGUANIDINE 64, 65
Sulphaguanidine tablets (F) (P)
    64
SULPHAMETHIZOLE 64, 66
Sulphamethizole tablets (F) (P)
    64
SULPHAMETHOXYPYRIDAZINE 64,
    66
Sulphamezathine (P) 64, 66
SULPHAPYRIDINE 64, 66
Sulphapyridine (P) 66
SULPHASALAZINE 28
SULPHATHIAZOLE 64, 66
Sulphatriad (P) 64, 66
SULPHAUREA 64, 66
SULPHINPYRAZONE 130, 195
SULPHUR (WITH OR WITHOUT
    RESORCINOL) (P+▲) 90-1
SULTHIAME 172-3, 194
Surem (P) 158
Sure-Shield Sur-Lax tablets (▲)
    30
Surgam (P) 126
Surmontil (P) 161, 163
Sustamycin (P) 62
Sweetex (▲) 57
Swiss Biofacial (▲) 93
Sylopal (P+▲) 20
Symmetrel (P) 70, 71, 174
Synalar (P) 97
Syndol (P) 192
Synflex (P) 178
Syntaris (P) 147
Syrup of Figs (▲) 30
Sytron (5 ml) (P+▲) 119

Tacitin (P) 154
Tagamet (P) 21
TALAMPICILLIN 60
Talpen (P) 60
Tampovagan stilboestrol and
  Lactic acid (P) 101
Tancolin (P+▲) 52
Tandacote (P) 127
Tandalgesic (P) 192
Tanderil (P) 127, 140
Tanderil Chloramphenicol (P)
  139, 140
Taractan (P) 168
Tarband (P+▲) 95–6
Tavegil (P) 149
TCP (▲) 93
  Antiseptic (▲) 151
Tears Naturale (P+▲) 143
Tedral (P) 43
  Expectorant (P) 51
  SA tablets (P) 43
Teejel (P+▲) 17
Tegretol (P) 171, 189
TEMAZEPAM 158
Temetex (P) 97
Temgesic and Temgesic sub-
  lingual (P) 182
Tenavoid (P) 156
Tensium (P) 155
Tenuate Dospan (P) 55
TERBUTALINE 41
TERFENADINE 149
Teronac (P) 56
Terra-Bron (P) 63
Terra-Cortril (P) 146
Terramycin (P) 62
Terramycin Ophthalmic Oint-
  ment with Polymyxin B
  Sulphate (P) 139
Tertroxin (P) 74
Testoral Sublings (P) 104
TESTOSTERONE 104
TETRABENAZINE 176
Tetrabid (P) 62
Tetrachel (P) 62
TETRACHLOROETHYLENE 107
Tetrachloroethylene capsules (F)
  (P+▲) 107
TETRACYCLINE 62, 83, 137, 145
Tetracycline (F) (P) 62
TETRACYCLINE AND NYSTATIN 63
Tetralysal (P) 62
Tetrex (P) 62
Thalazole (P) 64, 65
Thean (P+▲) 45
Theocontin continuus (P+▲)
  45
Theodrox (P+▲) 45
Theo-dur (P+▲) 45
Theograd (P+▲) 45
Theophorin (P+▲) 149
THEOPHYLLINATE 45
Theophylline (F) (P+▲) 45
THIABENDAZOLE 106, 107, 108
Thiazamide (P) 64, 66
THIETHYLPERAZINE 135
THIOPROPAZATE 168, 169
THIORIDAZINE 168
THYROXINE SODIUM 73–4
Thyroxine tablets (F) (P) 73–4
TIAPROFENIC ACID 126
TIMOLOL 143
Timoptol (P) 143
Tinaderm (P+▲) 85

Tineafax (P+▲) 85
Tinset (P) 149
Titralac (P+▲) 20
Tixylix (P+▲) 52
TOFENACIN 165, 166
Tofranil (P) 161, 162
Tolectin and Tolectin DS (P)
  126
TOLMETIN 126
TOLNAFTATE 85
Tonivitan A and D syrup (P+▲)
  122
Topal (P+▲) 18
Topilar (P) 97
Torbetol (P) 93
Torecan (P) 135
Tosmilen (P) 142
Trancopal (P) 154
Trancoprin (P) 192
Transvasin (P+▲) 125
Tranxene (P) 155
TRANYLCYPROMINE 165
TRAZODONE 161, 163, 165, 166
Tremonil (P) 176
TRETINOIN 92
Tri-Adcortyl Otic (P) 146
Triadol (P+▲) 178
TRIAMCINOLONE 16–17, 47
Triamcinolone (P) 47
TRIAMCINOLONE ACETONIDE 97
Triclocarban 83
Tridione (P) 173
TRIFLUOPERAZINE 43, 168, 169
Triludan (P) 149
TRIMEPRAZINE 88, 89
Trimeprazine tartrate (F)
  (P) 88, 89
TRIMETHOPRIM 137
TRIMIPRAMINE 161, 163
Trinordiol (P) 113
Triocos (P+▲) 148
Triogesic (P+▲) 148
Triominic (P+▲) 148
Triotussic (P+▲) 148
TRIPROLIDINE 149
Trisequens (P) 102
TROXIDONE 173
Tryptizol (P) 160, 161
TRYPTOPHAN 165, 166
Tuinal (P) 158
Turpentine Liniment (F) (P+▲)
  124
Tussifans Mixture (P+▲) 51

Ultradil (P) 97
Ultralanum (P) 97
Ultraproct (P) 36
UNDECENOATE 85
Uniflu+Gregovite C (P+▲)
  148
Unigesic (P+▲) 192
Unimycin (P) 62
UREA PREPARATIONS 95, 96
Urispas (P) 190
Urolucosil (P) 64, 66
Uromide (P) 64, 66
Uticillin (P) 59
Uvistat and Uvistat L (P+▲)
  86

Vaginal diaphragm (P+▲) 111
Valderma (▲) 93
Valium (P) 155
Valledrine (P) 52

Vallergan tablets and syrups (P)
  88, 89
Vallex (P) 51, 148
Valoid (P+▲) 133
Valrelease (P) 155
Vancocin (P) 28
VANCOMYCIN 28
Vanair (P+▲) 91
Vapex Inhalant (▲) 148
Variotin (P) 85
Vaseline (▲) 87
Vasocon A (P) 139
Vasogen (P+▲) 86
V-Cil-K (P) 60
Veganin (▲) 192
Velosef (P) 61
Venos Adult Formula (▲) 52
Venos Honey and Lemon (▲)
  52
Venos Original (▲) 52
Ventolin (P) 40
Veracolate (P+▲) 31
Veracur (P+▲) 94
Vermox (P) 106
Verrugon (P+▲) 94
Vertigon (P) 134–5
Vibramycin (P) 62
Vibrocil (P) 147
Vicks
  Cough Calmers (▲) 52
  Expectorant Cough Syrup (▲)
    51
  Formula 44 (▲) 52
  Inhaler (▲) 148
  Medinite (▲) 150
  Sinex Drops and Spray (▲)
    147
  Vaporub (▲) 148
VIDARABINE 137
Vidopen (P) 59
VILOXAZINE 161, 163, 194
Vimule (P+▲) 111
Vira-A (P) 137
Virormone (P) 99
Vi-Siblin (P+▲) 31
Vivalan (P) 161, 163
Voltarol (P) 126

Wartex (P+▲) 94
Water-repellent barrier (F)
  (P+▲) 87
Waxsol (P+▲) 144
Welldorm (P) 157
Wheat bran (F) (P+▲) 31
White Liniment (F) (P+▲) 124
Whitfield's ointment (P+▲) 83
Wigglesworth acne cream (▲)
  91

Xanax (P) 154
XANTHINE COMPOUNDS 45
Xerumenex (P+▲) 144
Xyloproct (P) 36

Yeast Vite (▲) 192
Yomesan (P+▲) 107–8

Zactipar (P) 192
Zactirin (P) 192
Zantac (P) 21
Zarontin (P) 173
Zelmid (P) 161, 164
ZIMELIDINE 161, 164
Zinamide (P) 67

Zinc and Adrenaline (P+▲) 143
Zinc and Coal Tar paste (F) (P+▲) 95–6
ZINC AND OIL PREPARATIONS 86–7

Zinc formulary preparations (F) (P+▲) 86–7, 91
Zincfrin (P+▲) 139
Zinc paste (F) (P+▲) 96
Zinc Paste Coal Tar bandage (F) (P+▲) 95–6

ZINC PREPARATIONS 88
Zinc sulphate (P+▲) 143
Zovirax (P) 70, 71, 137, 138
Zyloric (P) 129–30